Air Passages: Surviving Asthma Naturally

by Ted J. Cibik, ND, DMQ

Oak Tree Productions

2003

First Published in 2003

Publisher: Oak Tree Productions
                        825 Lovers Leap Rd.
                        Leechburg, PA 15656

Editors: Ted J. Cibik
                        LuAnn Cibik
                        Rebecca Pope
                        Geoff Litz
                        Dirce Johnson

Art/Photography: LuAnn Cibik

Copyright 2003, Ted. J. Cibik

Manufactured in the United States of America

ISBN: 0-9722853-0-X

Library of Congress catalog number:

All rights reserved. No part of this book may be used or reproduced in any manner whatsoever without the express written permission from the author, with the exception of brief quotations embodied within critical articles and reviews.

Disclaimer:
Qigong Medicine is not intended to replace orthodox medicine, but rather to complement it. The meditations, practices, techniques and prescriptions described herein are powerful and may be too mentally and physically demanding for some people. The readers should therefore use their own discretion and consult a Doctor of Medical Qigong therapy, acupuncturist, medical doctor, or mental health professional before engaging in these exercises and meditations.

DEDICATION

This book is dedicated to two of the most enlightened and
loving people I have ever met.
My parents, Joe and Leona,
who without their insight, courage and above all else faith
and love; I surely would be no more than a group of
alphabetic letters designating a small existence in time.

Thank you for the opportunity
to do great things
in this world
and to leave my mark.

Contents

DEDICATION

ACKNOWLEDGMENTS

INTRODUCTION
    Asthmatic's Survival Guide 10

CHAPTER 1
    Roots 15

CHAPTER 2:
    The Evolution of Asthma 26
Asthma Facts & Statistics 26
Food Allergens 27
Typical Non-allergenic Foods 27
Typical Allergy Triggers 28
    Food Additives 28
    Medicines 28
    Mold or Fungi 28
    Pollens 28
    Animal hair or fur 29
    Cockroaches 29
    Dust mites 29
    Alcohol 29
Irritants 30
    Smoke 30
    Chemicals 30
    Home Building Materials 30
    Exercise 31
    Weather 31
    MCS 31
    Stress and Anxiety 31
      Viruses or Colds 32
      Bacteria and Fungus 32
The Trigger 34

CHAPTER 3
    Anatomy 101, The Basic Stuff 35
The Lungs 35
The Brain 37
    The Brain Stem or the Reptilian Brain 37
    The Cerebellum or Limbic Brain 38
    The Cerebrum or Neocortex 39
    Beta Blocker Theory 40
Immune System Response 41
Immunoglobulin E 42
Mast Cells 43
Other Current Theories 43
The Skin 44
    Skin Inflammation & Allergic Itching 45

CHAPTER 4
The Theory of Hyperoxigenation 50
Three Regions of Breath 55
Blood 59
The Future 62

CHAPTER 5
Nutrition and Diet 63
The Truth about Diets 63
Eat to Live or Live to Eat 66
Macronutrient Ratio 68
Protein 69
Carbohydrates 69
Journaling 71
Chinese Diet Therapy 73
Sugar is a Food for Cancer 75
Low Glycemic Index Foods 76
Asthma and pH 77
Eating Patterns and pH Regulation 79
Breathing Patterns and pH Regulation 80
The Raw Food Diet for Asthma / Allergy Patients 81
Preparation of Food 82
Food Additives 83
    MSG 84
    Cochineal 84
    Yellow#5 85
    Red #3 85

CHAPTER 6
Detoxification and Supplementation 86
Creating a Detoxification Plan 86
Liver Stabilization Through Diet 89
Detoxification Bath and External Poultices 91
Immune Suppression Detoxification Diet 92
Protection from Common Tests Emanating Radiation 92
Antioxidants and Their Role in Fighting Free Radicals and Cancer 93
Antioxidants 93
    Vitamin E 95
    Vitamin E and Tocotrienol 95
    Vitamin C 96
    B Vitamins 96
    Supplements 97
    Alpha Lipoic Acid 97
    NAC N-Acetyl Cysteine 98
    L-Glutathione 98
    Melatonin 99
    Green Tea 99
    Grape Seed Extract 100
    Rooibos Tea 100
Photochemicals: Their Food Sources and Actions 100
Ginger 102
Litchi 102
Pumpkin 102
Phosphatidylserine 102
Forskolin 103

Localized Honey	103
Pycnogenol	104
Quercetin	104
Shark Liver Oil or Alkylglycerol	105
Borage Seed Oil	105
Zinc	106
Magnesium	106
Violence and Supplementation	107
Miscellaneous	107

CHAPTER 7

Exercise	108
Cardiovascular and Fat Burning Differences	112
Before Starting an Exercise Program	115
Water	115
Warm up First - ALWAYS!	117
Treadmill	118
A Treadmill Program for Asthmatics	118
Walk/Jog Program	119
Thermoregulate, in other words, Sweat!	120
Breathing Squats	121
Barbell Pullovers	124
Squat Kicks	125
Stomach and Abdominal Work	125
Creating a Super Strong Back that will Never Break	126
Jack Knives	128
Side to Side Jack Knives	128
Dips	128
Pushups!!!	129
Regular Breathing Pushups	130
Wide Breathing Pushups	130
Close Breathing Pushups	131
Fist Breathing Pushups	131
Finger Pushups	131
Triangle Breathing Pushups	132
Decline Breathing Pushups	132
Chinese Breathing Pushups	132
Stretching	133
Backstroke Stretch	134
Slap Sides	135
Front Stretch Kick	135
The Cat	135
Wag the Dog's Tail	136
Thread the Needle	136
Downward Facing Dog	137
Modified Fish	137
Pierce the Sky	138
Half Moon	138
Plies	139
Trembling Horse	139
Martial Arts Training	139
The Brief History of Inner Strength Martial Arts.	140

CHAPTER 8

Alternative Approaches	146
Why Alternative Approaches?	146

Sweat Therapy	*148*
Epsom Salts Baths	*150*
Hydrogen Peroxide Baths	*151*
Oatmeal Baths	*151*
Apple Cider Vinegar Baths	*151*
Baking Soda Baths	*152*
Coffee	*153*
Mucous	*153*
Saline Wash	*153*
Decline Purgation	*154*
Thumping	*154*
My Herbal Tincture	*156*

CHAPTER 9

Stress	*160*
Adrenal Burnout	*161*
Managing Your Stress	*163*
Chronobiology	*165*
Time Management	*167*

CHAPTER 10

The Mind	*170*
Meditation	*173*
Visualization	*177*
Breathing Techniques for Guided Visualization	*181*
Healing Meditations	*183*
Healing Meditations Preparation	*185*
The Four Fundamentals	*185*
White Tiger Meditation	*188*
Crashing Wave Meditation	*191*
Lung Expansion Meditation	*193*
Goals	*195*

CHAPTER 11

Pednisone & Albuterol	*197*
Serious Side Effects / LongTerm Effects	*199*
Infections	*199*
Chicken Pox	*199*
Drying Out	*200*
Call your doctor if you experience:	*201*
After long term use:	*201*
After you stop taking the drug, call your doctor immediately if you have:	*201*
Albuterol	*205*

CHAPTER 12

Chinese Medicine as Therapy	*207*
An Appointment with a Chinese Doctor	*208*
In the Beginning	*210*
Qi	*211*
Meridians	*212*
Yin and Yang	*215*
The Five Elements	*218*
The Taiji Pole	*219*
The Three Dan tians	*220*
Wei Chi Fields	*223*

Fear and the Kidneys 226
The Fear Factor and Asthma 227
Exacerbation of the Po Residing in the Lungs 228

CHAPTER 13
QiGong Exercise 230
Why QiGong Exercise? 231
Proof of QiGong Effectiveness 231
Health Benefits 232
QiGong Meets Western Exercise Science and Rehabilitation 233
QiGong Applications 236
Chinese Medical QiGong Exercise Prescription versus QiGong Exercise for Health 238
Chinese Medical QiGong 240

CHAPTER 14
Asthma QiGong 244
Getting Started 244
Centering 245
Breath Ratio Breathing Methods 245
The Three Steps of Practice 246
WuChi Posture 247
Purging 247
Tonify the Five Yin Organs 248
Preparation for Working the Yin Organs 248
Pull Down the Heavens QiGong Exercise: 248
QiGong Lung Exercise 249
QiGong Spleen Exercise 250
QiGong Kidney Exercise 251
QiGong Heart Exercise 252
QiGong Liver Exercise 252
Blend 252
Microcosmic orbit 253
Kwon Kong Stroking Beard 254
Asthma QiGong Preventative Maintenance Program 255

CHAPTER 15
Chinese Herbals 257
My Current Chinese Asthma Formula 260
Eczema and Chinese Herbals 261

FINAL THOUGHTS 262

FIVE PRECEPTS TO BECOMING A MASTER 263

BIBLIOGRAPHY 264

RESOURCES FROM INNER STRENGTH
Videotapes 267
    Asthma QiGong: Your Self Defense for Asthma 267
    Your Self Defense for Stress 267
CDS 267
    Medical QiGong for the 21st Century 267

ABOUT THE AUTHOR 269

Acknowledgments

All experiences are cumulative and like life, many people have allowed me to make this book happen.

I would first like to thank my beautiful wife, LuAnn, for her constant support, love, and encouragement and for allowing me to bathe in her angelic presence. I would also like to thank her for her amazing technical ability, as she took many of the photos in this book and I greatly appreciate her technical skill and insight in arranging the graphics. Thank you for your valuable advice on many drafts of this book.

I am also extremely grateful and indebted to Dr. Jerry Alan Johnson for his wisdom, kindness and his teaching of Medical Qigong and Chinese medicine. His vision and willingness to share will always be remembered.

I am also grateful to Jeffrey Yuen, whose teachings are timeless and have allowed me to expand my horizons in the art of Chinese Medicine.

I wish to thank Rebecca Pope, the senior editor of this manuscript, who unselfishly gave her valuable time and expertise in editing so that I would look good. Thank you for your investment in this project.

A warm thanks to Phyllis Framel, whose kindness in editing will not be forgotten.

A special thanks to Jeff Litz, whose keen editing eyes prevented me from many embarrassing moments of readership.

I would like to express my gratitude to Dirce Johnson, whose insight and confidence in this project as well as many hours of research are appreciated.

Finally, to Max who was with me the entire time I wrote this book and who is deeply missed, but never forgotten.

INTRODUCTION

Surviving Asthma Naturally

I believe in the things that I am about to write here. Moreover, I practice to this day the things I write here. No, I am not the poetic philosopher or a medical doctor; rather, these things come from my experience, my life, my insight, and my very heart and soul.

The one attribute I knew I had from a very small child was a mindset of …*"that no matter what…there was always another option…(I) you just haven't thought of it yet"*. Another way of looking at this is that you never give up trying. There has been a lot written about the attribute of persistence. Persistence is the way sentient being's conquer their ills. The mind is an incredible tool. Like any tool, your mind can be utilized for good, for bad, for the right way and for the wrong way; it can make your work easier, or it can make it twice as hard. For people with chronic illness and pain, their only salvation is persistence. I know of very few people who obtain immediate relief from their serious illnesses. Many times, it is a long journey filled with crushed hopes and disappointments before the goal of health is reached.

Being martial or warlike is one way you can deal with illness. After all, this is your war, your battle with your personal disease. Take it personally; make up your mind that you will take responsibility for the war, like the general, andthat only death will make you stop trying. No one else can better understand your disease than you can. Therefore, no one can be the true general of the war other than you. You must lead with controlled and channeled fear, and you must persist, for only then will there be peace in your soul.

Martial arts/meditation helped me so much in my mindset to battle my ailments that I must write about it in hopes that it helps someone else. Illness, injury, life-threatening disease - this is all warfare. You must approach it like warfare and accept nothing less than victory. Battles may be lost. Setbacks are many. Unforeseen problems do arise, but in the end you must win. You must conquer. This is your life and you, my friend, are responsible for the battle and the courage to do battle. Dying is nothing to be ashamed of. Death is not a punishment for failing. Quitting is punishment for failing. The samurai of Japan were not afraid to die by honor, or for what they believed in. You must believe in yourself and forgive yourself for being human and for the mistakes and setbacks that being human entails. Being perfect is not human.

It is amazing how powerful the mind is. It can change your entire being. It can save your life or take it away. Life is hard for everyone; we just don't know what kind of suffering other people are going through. We have a tendency to judge based on our perceptions, rather than from the world of the other person. Jesus, Budda, and Wen-shu, tried to make us aware of this and so did many other enlightened beings. Many times the mental anguish far surpasses the physical. This was true in my case, and I am positive it is true for many others.

The difficult task is to gain control of the mind and thereby the emotions that are a by-product of our thought patterns. Many times negative thinking is so circular that we never realize how often we think the same thoughts, organized in different ways. We often have a tendency to think in simular patterns that can be negative or positive or a combination of both. The point is, we think the same thought over and over again with little room for deviation. The first step in thinking outside the box is to acknowledge that we are thinking the same thoughts repeatedly.

Now that you have acknowledged that your thoughts are repeating, you must have the courage to let your mind and intuition go, to live on the edge of uncertainty, and to accept new ideas with faith and trust without attachment to the outcome. Do this knowing that you will learn much on the way that will contribute to your final destination.

The twenty-first century is an unprecedented time of available information. Many people often times categorize therapies such as mine as alternative therapy. Actually, the kind of treatment described in this book and the driving force in saving my life is one of the original healing modalities; it dates back almost 8,000 ago to the area known as the Hawaiian Islands. This type of treatment was called Fu Shi, and later became a popular treatment method that spread to China, including Tibet. It is almost funny that we have coined the phrases "alternative treatment" or "new age" for this modality of healing. Breathing therapies have existed in a formalized sense since man became willing to treat and help his fellow man. Since breathing is so fundamental to life and thereby health, it is only natural that man would develop therapies surrounding that concept.

One thing I have observed in the past is the "us" or "them" mentality. Some allopathic physicians did not want to share the responsibility of combining western science with so-called alternative methods. Many believed that drugs and surgery could cure everything. On the other side of the fence are the holistic or alternative medicine people who many times suggest that allopathic physicians are not needed. Holistic practitioners feel that their system is complete and the allopathic physicians and therapists think theirs is complete. Neither is correct, especially in the case of asthma. Rescue drug remedies are definitely needed. Preventative therapy is definitely needed; including breathing therapies! The two camps must learn and are finally learning to work together. Ultimately, it is the asthma consumer's responsibility to become educated, to experiment, and to persevere in taking responsibility for their own health.

Why do I want to write a book in the first place, I thought? I do not have the time. I do not have the money to publish it and what if nobody reads the darn thing? That will really make me feel like I wasted my time and energy, I kept thinking to myself. Then I read a statistic. A research group in North Dakota found that asthmatics who wrote about the stressful events in their lives improved their breathing capacity by almost 20 percent! "Darn, my whole life has been stressful, I ought to be able to increase that number to 80% at least," I thought! So my journey began into the wonderful world of typing, misspelling words, and finding the time to compose them. I blocked off the time on my calendar, rearranged my work day, got up earlier and went to bed late.

This book is going to be different I vowed. I want it to be an owner's manual for asthmatics. I am not a world renowned internist or pediatrician, nor did I graduate from Harvard with honors, but I live day to day with asthma and I have learned "tricks" along the way to help me live a normal (I use that word with caution) life.

This book will outline everything I have researched and learned over the last 35 years to help myself. Some of these techniques you may already know, some you may have never heard of, and some are of my own creation. They have one thing in common, though, they work for me and they may work for you, too. I sometimes will use "asthma" or "allergies" in singular context, but usually I mean them as one entity.

I am thankful I am an asthmatic. Having the asthma and allergies has carved a very unique individual (me) in this world and showed me some of the most fundamental truths about living and life that one could ever experience. Asthma has made me the physical, mental and spiritual man I am today. I am proud to admit that. For twenty or so years I would never admit I had asthma. It was a "disease". It was something that separated me out from the other normal kids and, later, adults. Now, I have an opportunity to share my thoughts and ideas with people and, in my heart, I hope to help them in a way that I wished that someone could have helped me when I was young.

I also am one of these people that always wanted someone to get to the point. "Forget the sales pitch, the fluff, get to the point" I would always scream in my head. Therefore, I hope that I get to the point with my "tricks". After my tricks are presented, I will try to verify and support them scientifically, epidemiologically, empirically, and with my own version of logic, which I have been told is quite novel (Pun intended).

This will hopefully be a book about self-discovery for you and I both. I will get to remember things long forgotten and suppressed, and you may have insight into why you thought or felt certain ways. I don't expect you to agree with everything in this book, nor can I claim that for all of my techniques are scientifically proven to work on the vast majority of people. Everything in this book has helped me and hundreds of my clients, and I hope you will keep an open mind to try these methods so that I may be able to help you too.

I think asthmatics, or anyone who faces life-threatening circumstances can evolve into appreciative thinkers who make a giant step toward being self-actualized or enlightened beings. It does not matter what your biological age is, as children can become painfully aware of intense responsibility at a young age. Actually, I don't know if we evolve or are pushed into this line of thinking by survival mechanisms. I guess this sounds a little condescending, but I think people like us appreciate the simple things in life to an enhanced degree. For people like us, the warmth of the sun and the beauty of the colors of the sky, the companionship and laughter of a close friend, the beauty of single mindfulness of thought, all become the highlights of a day. This is because you know that tomorrow can be the last day, or can be miserable beyond comprehension and description. In that moment of misery, all you can concentrate on is your survival, on trying to heal your body again and stabilizing your mind into being positive.

It is my hope that this book becomes your survival kit, your Bible, and your inspiration for taking control again of your mind and body and thereby your health.

Ted J. Cibik

September, 2003

CHAPTER 1
Roots

This is the hardest chapter to write so I am beginning with it. I have always been that way, doing the hardest part first. Whether this is a product of nature or nurture, I am not sure. I often wonder how much my asthma and allergies have shaped my personality, my emotions, my drive and tenacity as well as my viewpoints and all the qualities that make up "Ted". I guess I will never truly know how my life would have been different if I had not had asthma and allergies. I hope in some small way, after someone reads my story, it will help at least one person somewhere. If it does, then I will be happy. This will be hard, as it forces me to think of things I have not had to dwell on in years. Painful memories. Life was tough for me as a kid. I just wanted to be "like everyone else". Now as an adult, I wonder what I really wanted, as I no longer desire to be like anyone else.

The year was 1964. Although I do not remember everything, just fragments of what happened, my parents fill in the gaps. It all started when my mother was feeding me wheat cereal one day. My mother can't recall that I ever had a problem with allergies before. However, on this day my face swelled almost instantly and I began coughing and gasping for air. I was having an anaphylactic reaction. Back in the 60's, of course, there was no home injectable kit of epinephrine to administer. My parents rushed me to the hospital. My father said he didn't want to wait for the ambulance (we lived back on a very windy country road). My father, who to this day is one of the best drivers I know, said he was speeding about 80 to 90 miles per hour in some areas. My mother was holding me in the front seat of the car. Remember, this is before seat belts. I remember her telling me that my lips and fingers were a deep blue color from lack of oxygen.

When we got to the hospital, I do remember them placing me in an oxygen tent. The plastic covering of this thing distorted my view from the inside, and with all these strangers yelling and running around, I can remember the panic I felt being separated from my parents . This obviously doesn't help someone with asthma! The sound also was very frightening a whooshing sound that muffled everything. I also remember that the oxygen tent seemed to make it harder to breath the exact opposite of what it was supposed to do. I remember my mother crawling in the oxygen tent with me to calm me down. I felt a sense of peace. After that, I do not remember much about the treatment, but my mother later filled in the gaps for me.

Apparently, the doctors eventually diagnosed me with severe asthma and were calling in a respiratory specialist. At this point, I was slipping in and out of consciousness, although I maintained eye contact with my mother and father. My asthma attack was now on its third day and my body was severely weak, dehydrated, and fatigued from trying to squeeze air into my lungs. The physicians thought a massive heart attack was imminent. I still was conscious and moving, though rather slowly. In hindsight, I now know from my adult asthma attacks, that instinctively I was conserving all my energy to focus on breathing. The doctors approached my parents and suggested that they may want to contact a priest because it could be a matter of hours before I died. My parents, of course, still had hope for me.

The physician in charge of my case had searched throughout the world for asthma cases that were this severe and for similar complications. He found none. It was at that point that collectively the doctors came up with a long shot. The specialist they called in had a radical idea that had never been attempted before. He wanted to paralyze my body to allow my heart muscle to recuperate long enough so that I would not go into cardiac arrest or "stroke out". The drug they were going to use was called Curare, a plant (now drug) from South America. South American Indians rub Curare onto spears and darts in blowguns, then shoot their animal prey, usually monkeys, which then fall out of trees from paralysis to be clubbed to death.

Curare was administered to me, although when signing the consent forms, my parents were made aware that the doctors had no concept of how much to use on a human being -let alone in a state of breakdown- and that there were no completed clinical trials on Curare. They were also told that even if I survived this bout, that my long-term survival was minimal at best. Unfortunately, or fortunately (who is to say at this point), the physician administered far too much of the paralyzing drug. Later we learned that six times the lethal dose was intravenously infused into my body.

My body became totally paralyzed for three days, first starting with my face, progressing to my neck, inhibiting my ability to swallow or lift my head and finally paralyzing my diaphragm. Since the heart is a muscle, my heart became paralyzed eventually as well. No movement was recorded. Primitive breathing apparatus was used to sustain oxygen delivery. They even used artificial tears for my eyes so they would not dry out. My body had completely shut down all voluntary and involuntary movement that they could record via apparatus. The physicians had never seen such a reaction and were clueless what to do. Clinically I was pronounced dead.

My Catholic parents called in a priest to give me last rites at 4 am. I am sure that this is the hardest thing in the world for a parent to do. All they had was their faith in God, as the doctors were perplexed, confused and walking in uncharted territory of paralysis and drug interaction and my body's own state of breakdown.

By the fourth day I had "miraculously" regained consciousness. The medical records are incomplete at best, as I have tried to locate them, but apparently I died. No one knows for sure, but from reports in JAMA (yes, I was written up as a case study but many details were left out) and from talking with the physicians in charge at the time, they believe I was dead for 15 minutes before life signs came back. When I did regain consciousness everyone proclaimed it a miracle, even the doctors. For the next several days, my parents and I were bombarded with questions from physicians, psychologists, clergy and everyone else who was interested in what happens with life-after-death issues.

The only thing I kept repeating was, "There was a beautiful lady who talked so nice to me" and that "I wasn't scared at all". It was also apparent that while I was gone I did not seem to cry or miss my parents. It was not documented that I reported experiencing anything such as a tunnel or a white room like many of the other people who have clinically died and returned to report what they have seen. Throughout the rest of my childhood, I could remember certain events that took place in that time warp of death and revival.

Later as an teeneage and adult, I often speculated about my sensory experience of that moment as I am still able to remember certain events that took place on my journey to "the other side". But this will be the focus of another book entirely!

One thing I only recently realized while researching this book is that I frequently wake at night at the exact same time that I died in the hospital (3:40 am), and I have for as long as I can remember.

If you spend enough time in hospitals, you naturally will see people "disappear"' from the hospital ward. At least that is one thought I used to have. The kids I would talk to during the day and at night were all at once gone. Some of the kids I thought were taken home by their parents. I instinctively knew that others had something wrong with them before they "disappeared". The scary thing is that I always knew when they were going to expire. I think that was the most frightening thing as a child in a hospital. The treatments were not as frightening, because you had a nurse and your parents to explain what was going to happen. However, the unknown is always terrifying, even for adults, let alone children. I somehow knew that the dying children were happier than anyone could imagine, but I remember feeling so sorry for their parents. I could not at this young age explain to them about what happened to children who die. I just knew from my experience that death for children is not frightening, not painful, but a joyous event that children instinctively understand and comprehend.

Most of my childhood I remember finishing the school year in hospitals around the country. My parents were always reading and researching about my conditions. They would try most anything. Unfortunately, I was one of the ten worst asthma cases ever recorded, according to what doctors told my parents at that time. Most hospitals did not have the drugs or technology at that time to treat such extreme conditions.

Standard medications and therapies did not heal my skin, nor did they allow me to breathe better. My parents were told to prepare for the fact that I would most likely die from a multitude of complications before the age of 18. Two scenarios were given to me: either my immune system would break down so far that I would succumb to massive infection, or my heart, after constant abuse of asthma attack after asthma attack, would fall victim to a massive heart attack or possible stroke. Some of my earlier asthma attacks would last in varying degrees of breathlessness for three to six days.

Because my skin was constantly itchy and I had a rash all over my body, even in my scalp, it was a constant battle to keep me clean from infection. I was prescribed prednisone (more on that later) but after several years of use, that drug also compromised my immune system and added to my constant infections. I can remember constantly smelling pus from where scratches became infected and the boils on my skin . This happened up until I was about 14. I can remember how conscious I was even at the age of 10 and 12 of how other people would look at me because of the way my skin looked. I remember too how others looked at my parents as if they were neglectful! This would make me mad as hell, because I could see the expressions in their eyes. How dare they judge us, I used to think, when they don't even have a clue about the circumstances.

My parents did not try to make me live in a bubble; they wanted me to experience a little of life's pleasures such as playing outside, building tree-houses and chasing my dog around the yard. When I was four, my parents retrofitted an old farm house on top of a mountain with state-of-the-art environmental controls, and we moved away from the dampness of the valley. My parents knew that by the time I was 10, I had the mental outlook of an adult when it came to judging what I could or could not do without repercussions. I was responsible for taking my medications and knowing exactly how to take them. At that time in my life, I could tell you all the contraindications of each pill, what each was used for, dosages for various patients and all common uses of that medication. I had researched the biology and explored the anatomy and physiology of the lungs in my constant love of reading and books.

My parents wanted me to go to public school to learn how to socialize and have as normal an upbringing as possible. Going to school was exhausting because I itched constantly and wheezed just in normal activities, let alone when trying to run and play at recess, which I couldn't do. I can remember how everything would itch at once, even the inside of my ears, mouth and eyes. The itch always felt deep, beneath the skin and in the very core of my body itself.

Throughout the school day I used the Zen meditation I had learned (more on that later) to try to put myself in another place so that I didn't feel the itch and the panic of not getting enough air. By the time the school day was over, I was mentally exhausted from concentrating so deeply on not constantly scratching and on calming myself to get my air, not to mention trying to absorb my school work. I used to have to split myself into two persons almost, one to listen to the teacher and the other to keep myself from becoming overwhelmed with my afflictions. I miraculously had good grades in school as it came rather easy for me.

Along with the numerous infections came intense fevers. I recall one time having been itchy for weeks because I was trying to play in the grass with my dog. My skin was all broken out with large open wounds that bled and were full of pus. It should be understood that my parents had taken me to the doctors' and I was taking antibiotics again, but they were not appearing to help as they normally did. I remember burning up one day on the couch and the fever seemed to come on all at once. My vision was starting to blur and that is when I became scared and told my parents to get me to the hospital because something was wrong with me. They knew how I hated to go there, so they knew this must be serious.

My temperature was 105 and climbing. The doctors had me sitting naked in a bathtub loaded with ice while intravenous fluids dripped into me. The intravenous needle was in an odd place, I remember, between my knuckles. I had to stay in the ice bath for two days and nights, and was only allowed to come out of the bathtub occasionally to un-cramp my body. Finally, the fever broke.

Different events release different kinds of energy and/or emotions in people. I remember the frustration of the physicians with me the most. Even in my adolescent years, I could sense their confusion and frustration when they would talk to me and my parents about what they were going to try on me next. Once I was hospitalized for a severe allergic reaction on my skin that lead to hives, rash, intense itching and an extreme fire and heat that manifested itself as redness from my head to toes. The doctors could not isolate the cause, except that I was allergic to "everything". This lead to another serious staph infection. After hospitalization, the infection was cleared with another antibiotic drip. I was kept in the hospital for more study and I continued to lose weight.

My pediatrician at the time came up with a very novel and holistic idea.....fasting. The concept of fasting has been around since man wanted to purge himself of toxins whether that was a spiritual toxin, mental or physical, but was unheard of in Western mainstream hospitals at this time. The purpose of this 9-day fast without food or drink was to disperse all the allergens out of my body. The only thing I was allowed to consume was black tea with a little sugar and water. The hardest part was not having any food, but rather was lying in bed with nothing to do all day and thinking about food because I could not have any. I can remember the smell of delicious hospital food being served on the carts to other patients (yes, I was a little delirious). I was incredibly weak at the end of the seventh day, although I was confined to bed rest. Most activities were a chore, the simple act of lifting my head became an effort. By the ninth day, when they started to reintroduce foods one by one, I was almost lifeless. My skin did clear, however. In hindsight, I see that I was not exposed to any dust or pollen from the outside, or to any internal allergens from ingestion of anything that could possibly have a reaction. Of course, my skin cleared.

Three months later, I was still hospitalized and still having problems with my skin allergies and asthma. Regardless of the fact that I only ate turkey, beets and rye bread, I was still on constant prednisone, Marax and several other medications, and for the most part in a sterile hospital environment (free of dust, pollen etc.). The next therapy they tried was for me to lie out in the sun for increasing amounts of time to "dry up" the allergies on my skin. This only exacerbated my symptoms and my skin became more inflamed and itchy either from the heat of the sun or the sun's rays itself. It was never determined which. The consequences of this experiment was more prednisone, and eventually my skin did clear. I was then released from hospital care and the doctors said that there was nothing further they could do.

I could not live hospitalized like this they realized. For the next several years all I lived on was turkey, rice, beets and occasionally a slice of rye bread. These were the only foods I could tolerate, and the doctors would not, as they would today, permit a rotation diet. No breads, chocolate, eggs, pasta, citrus (oranges, limes grapefruits, etc.), potatoes, corn, peas, chicken or poultry, spices, milk, or anything artificially colored, flavored or added were allowed at all. I was forbidden to play in the grass, be around any animals with hair or fur, to be in any dusty areas, or to wear clothing made of wool. I was required to stay indoors most of the time other than winter, when most of the pollen had died off.

I can remember going shopping for school clothes when I was a kid. I would always choose dark colors. The reason was that dark colors did not show the blood as well as lighter colors did. My skin had a habit of breaking open, splitting into wide cracks that would be an inch long, and bleed during activity. The activity did not have to be strenuous. It could be something as simple as getting out of a chair or walking down the hall. This was, needless to say, very embarrassing to me as it was difficult to explain to school children, let alone physicians.

I can also remember the doctors saying that the ocean would be good for my skin as the salt water would be healing to my open wounds. On several occasions my parents would go to the ocean shore and try to get me to walk in to the ocean. I loved the ocean, with its primordial sound of crashing waves and power. I hated the way the ocean felt on my skin though. Since the first layer of my skin was always rubbed raw and bleeding, cracked, itching and peeling anyway, the salt water was extremely painful and "burned" my skin like a rug burn that had salt rubbed into it.

This was most of my asthmatic childhood as I remember it. The medical part just seemed to repeat itself over and over. The hospital visits and the home remedies my parents designed to make me comfortable consumed my life. Life was about just being able to get through the day and putting on a mask for the rest of the world to see, so they would not judge or see me any differently than other children in school or activities.

The other part of my life, my personal life as opposed to my medical life, was far different. I knew from very young age that I must take control of my life, if I was to have one. At age 5, I began to beg my parents to allow me to take martial arts lessons. Just before I turned 6, they finally gave me the okay and I started Jiu-Jitsu. The instructor was kindly and huge. He had learned and trained in martial arts in Japan and was a staunch traditionalist in his teachings. I was most intrigued by his meditation techniques because meditation is a breathing method, and God knows I needed to learn how to breathe better. I instinctively knew that this was the right path for me and that I had to learn more about it. Later, I discovered that what I was learning from my Jiu-Jitsu instructor was Zen meditation. I loved Zen meditation as much as I loved learning how to do forward rolls and breakfalls. Strange, I know, but my world was different from the word "go" anyway.

In the early sixties, children did not commonly do martial arts as they do today. The training was much different then and so was the focus of the training. Most of the people who trained were men from the military and it was very physical. I enjoyed the discipline of the martial arts, the philosophy of self control taught by teachers, and the discipline's stress on self-dependence These are important to me to this day.

In addition to my martial arts training, at around age 12, I began reading anything I could get my hands that was about alternative treatment for allergies and asthma (I began reading when I was 4). Most of these books were pretty dry textbooks and college texts, as I was determined to outlive my life expectancy of 18! I read American Indian treatments, Chinese treatments, and Indian (Ayurvedic) treatments. I read about any culture that had something to say. My parents never denied me a book, no matter what the cost. They knew I would read it, but they didn't know I would study it. They also encouraged me by buying various nutritional supplements, herbs, or ingredients that I needed to test out a new theory of mine.

It was around twelve that I also discovered TM (Transcendental Meditation). A cousin who learned it in college taught it to me. I began to incorporate this breathing method into my everyday practice. A lot of what I did after that came out of my own mind, imagination and instincts, as I did not have a mentor every time I practiced and I had learned what I considered just basics. I was sure that both of these methods (Zen and TM) were lifetime endeavors.

By the time I was a teenager, I was starting to pull theories of mine together and had come up with a multicultural healing program that I would follow. Ideas about nutrition, meditation, breathing therapies, herbals, exercise and martial arts all were starting to gel into a game plan that I would have to follow to keep myself alive. I still used my doctor's advice, but as the physician who was the head of pediatrics at this hospital told my parents "you have gone through so much, have tried so much, lived with it day to day, you are the experts, not us"!

Later, this same doctor asked me to speak to graduating medical students to complete their education from a patient's perspective. After my doctor relayed my story to them, a round table of interns asked me random questions. I can remember being amazed at what questions they asked me, but I can also remember several of the graduates crying when they heard my story. I told them about what various therapies felt like, and about what it was like to live as a severe asthmatic. Their response and emotional reaction amazed and shocked me as a teenager, since I had always believed growing up that everyone goes through his or her own trials and tribulations. I believe, even to this day, that we all have things that shape us and that we must look for the good in it all and focus on that aspect of living.

I continued through my teenage years to research and develop my esoteric and eclectic modalities of treatment for myself. I must confess, that sometimes I think everyone knows all of this material. They have to, in order to survive! Then an awakening will come as I talk with a client and I realize that many people do not think on the same plane as I do. What I understand as instinct, sometimes needs to be explained or clarified to them.

I have had some wonderful teachers in my life, starting of course with my parents. My educational path has been a unique and unconventional one at best. I became a student at age five when I knew that I must take control of my health and my life. Since then it has been a constant search for knowledge through books, speaking with other health professionals, and of course, studying with those I call masters of their craft in healthcare.

My studies have taken both a traditional and untraditional paths. Yes, I have a traditional college education, but many of the things that helped me most were not taught in traditional schools or certification courses as they are today. After reading or hearing about a particular teacher or mentor, I would call or write to him or her and ask if I could train with them and pick their brain for a period of time. Instead of going to Disney and/or the beach to relax on vacation, these kinds of internships gratified my insatiable quest for knowledge and understanding.

I always believed that to truly understand something you must experience it, practice it, then rethink and rework it and then practice it some more. Rather than just memorize something for a test and then forget it, I always chose to learn and incorporate that knowledge into my own schemata.

Now to bring the focus back to the present. Stories are always more pleasant when they have a happy ending. I have more than tripled my predicted life expectancy, and have no intention of stopping soon. I do not know what the ending will be yet, but I do know that I have found my calling. I thoroughly enjoy helping people find the answers for a better quality of life through health, education and intuitive awakening.

This book presents a different approach to treating asthma, my approach from living and breathing with asthma all my life. As Surgeon General David Hatcher, MD was quoted as saying in a New York Times article, "Asthma is one area in which we are going in the wrong direction."[1]

My sincere wish is that everyone who reads this book comes away with something. That something may be different for each reader, but I pray that on some plane, they have a greater understanding, even if it is intuitive rather than tangible. In any event, writing this book has helped me to recapture my roots and what has shaped me. Perhaps you may want to do the same in your own journaling therapy.

1. Stollberg,S.G. *Poor fight baffling surge in asthma. The New York Times*, October 18, 1999

CHAPTER 2:

The Evolution of Asthma

"You cannot solve a problem with the same mind that created it"
- Albert Einstein

Asthma Facts & Statistics

The percentage of children acquiring asthma has doubled in 2 decades! It affects a little over 17 million people in the United States alone with young children being the most at risk. Reported cases of children with asthma have increased over 160% since 1980 according to the Centers for Disease Control and Prevention. For children, it is the number one cause of hospitalization in the United States and the sixth ranking cause of hospitalization overall.

The number of allergic sufferers is staggering. Over 50 million people worldwide (and growing) are afflicted with allergies which lead to such diseases as asthma, dermatitis, sinusitis, and rhinitis. Allergies are the sixth leading cause of disease in the United States and cost the healthcare system over $18 billion dollars per year!

If we could measure or tabulate misery in the United States, think of all the coughing, sneezing, wheezing, watery eyes, fatigue, itching and inflammation endured on a daily basis. Not only is this annoying, but it can cause lost productivity in school and work. It is estimated that over 5,000 people die annually from asthma.

Let's look at what causes asthma and the allergic reactions that can hasten asthma attacks. Asthma and allergies often go hand in hand. Of the children and adults I have talked to who have both, with one more severe than the other. A few of us have both severe asthma and allergies. Nevertheless, what actually happens?

First, there has to be a trigger. Something internally or externally has to trigger the actual responses in the body that cause the classic asthma attack. The classic asthma attack consists of muscle spasm, wheezing, tightness in the chest, excess mucous, fatigue, and coughing. I was one who never coughed during my asthma attacks, although most asthmatics I know do this. It just proves that each person reacts a little differently.

There are several types of triggers. Probably the most common are allergens. The list of allergens is endless because they vary from person to person. The following are common allergens that the majority of the population seems to have sensitivity to.

Food Allergens

In all my years of having allergies and meeting hundreds of other allergic people, I have come to realize that one can develop an allergy to almost any food. However, I have found that certain foods have a stronger history of causing reactions than most. They are: peanuts, wheat; eggs, milk (although goat's milk can sometimes be a good alternative), tomatoes and all tomato paste sauces, citrus (oranges), shellfish family (such as shrimp), and mustard.

Actually, it is probably easier to complete a list of safe foods, than to list all foods that a person could be allergic to.

Typical Non-allergenic Foods

Below is a partial list of foods within each nutritional category that are generally safe. It is a pretty short list at best, and even these can be suspect.

> Proteins - *Lamb, turkey, wild rabbit or most wild animals such as deer (venison)*
>
> Carbohydrates - *rice, beets, buckwheat (not related to wheat family), squash, cauliflower, sweet potatoes, cranberries, and apples.*
>
> Fats – *olive oil.*

Beware of Celiac disease (inflammation of the small intestine) or as it is now called gluten intolerance which causes diarrhea and nutritional and vitamin deficienes. This condition was the first sign to me that I had allergies to food. In addition, many times bowel or gastric discomfort is a sign the body gives to alert to allergic response. Most grains, including wheat, buckwheat and even corn can be a source of problems. Safe bets here are millet and rice. An interesting note is that raw garlic, when eaten with grains that cause sensitivity, can reduce the inflammation process and many times stop it all together!

Typical Allergy Triggers

A further list of allergen suspects would include:

Food Additives

Monosodium glutamate (MSG), additives and preservatives, dyes and sulfites (more on this later).

Medicines

Individual reactions may vary, but, for example, penicillin may cause some people to react, as well as several of the more powerful antibiotics such as Cipro. Antibiotics and antitetanus injections can cause anaphylactic shock. Beware of aspirin (or other NSAIDS) as they can induce asthma as well.

Mold or fungi

Molds are found indoors and outdoors. Many of us have heard of mildew in basements and in the bathroom or bread mold, but there are many other varieties. The funny brown color on the old plastic shower curtain is mold and can cause problems for asthmatics as well as skin allergies. Molds are microscopic fungi that live off their hosts to survive. That pile of compost that you spread on the garden or any other organic material for planting may contain enough mold spores to create an allergic reaction for you. Cutting down dense brush, mowing high grass or cleaning out that dark corner of your basement will probably disperse mold spores. I know from living on the farm that when the time for making hay and thrashing wheat arrived you could smell and feel the allergens in the air, many of which were mold spores.

Pollens

Here is a list that could go on forever. Tree pollen such as oak, maple or pine, or the pollen of your favorite flower could be causing your congestion, wheezing, and stuffy nose. Since pollens are air born and can travel miles, the entire geographic area becomes suspect. Grasses, shrubs and indoor plants can all contribute to peoples' allergies and therefore their asthma. Even if you sailed out into the middle of the Atlantic Ocean, there would still be pollen in the air.

Animal hair or fur

Your favorite pet with its long hair, or even short, could be causing you grief. Many times it is not the hair or fur itself, but the dander that the animal naturally sheds and which accumulates in the carpet, coach, pillows and throw rugs that is the culprit. Cats are more problematic for asthma sufferers than dogs as they produce more allergin from their constant grooming. Salivary protein is the main culprit in cats and has been found in homes where cats don't even exist!

Cockroaches

Cockroaches may not necessarily be in your living quarters, but in apartments, the food left by a neighbor who moved out may be a welcome home to these annoying creatures. Their dried feces can blow through air conditioning and heating ducts and create an invisible problem for you.

Dust mites

Dust mites can affect just about all of the people who have allergies. Your best defense against them is prevention. Keep the house below a relative humidity of 45%. Dust mites cannot live in such an environment, and the active ones will die. The inactive mites, however, will remain dormant and revive if the relative humidity rises above 55%.

Alcohol

In addition, I have heard of more and more people becoming allergic to beer and alcohol, perhaps due to the additives, preservatives, and pesticides used to growing grain, malt and hops. Be aware of herbal tinctures and homeopathic remedies that contain alcohol especially if you are allergic to corn, since that is what grain alcohol is largely derived from.

Irritants:

Another type of trigger for asthma/allergy attacks is an irritant.

Smoke

This includes cigarette, cigar and pipe smoke either firsthand or secondhand. Tobacco of all varieties contains over 4,000 chemicals in its smoke and some of these are carcinogens that can inhibit the red blood cells ability to carry life-giving oxygen. Needles to say, this is very dangerous for an asthmatic or anyone with breathing disorders!

In addition, burning leaves, fireplaces, candles and invisible vapors from ammonia and other chemical products such as cleaning supplies are problematic.

Chemicals

Perfume and cologne, tobacco (again first or second hand), insecticides, fresh paint smells, automobile exhaust (gas or diesel), household cleaning products, synthetic fabrics, aerosol air freshener, even plastics and inks!

Never mix cleaning products together, as the vapors can be harmful or even fatal. Smog, air pollution and space heaters can all be problematic.

Home Building Materials

Particleboard, plywood, fumes from indoor carpet pad and some rugs, paints (those without mold preventative), paint thinners and wood stains, fiberglass insulation, and polyurethane sealants. If you are wallpapering, make sure that you use mold-free wallpaper paste.

Exercise

Exercise induced asthma has received more publicity lately with professional athletes and Olympians who admit they have asthma yet still actively compete and compete well. A theory of mine is that it is not the exercise itself, but the deeper breathing of allergens that causes some of the exercise-induced attacks.

Weather

Biometeorology is the study of weather and climate changes that affect the human body's ability to adapt to these changes. Extreme cold or humidity or even a drastic fluctuation in the barometric pressure can bring on symptoms of asthma. For example, Spring and Summer thunderstorms have been shown to increase hospitalization of asthma patients; also the itch from eczema can become exacerbated by the change in air temperature.

Multiple Chemical Sensitivity

Multiple chemical sensitivity (MCS) is a by-product of the many chemical products and their by-products that we mass-produce today. Just about everything we produce, especially from petrochemicals, is linked to some sort of sensitivity in at least part of the population. In fact, the Labor Institute has found enough justification to print a 95-page booklet (almost a book) on Multiple Chemical Sensitivities at Work, to educate consumers. (New York, The Labor Institute, 1993)

Stress and Anxiety

In my experience, stress can exacerbate asthma. That is a fact I have been telling physicians for 20 years, but they always said "there is no proof of that." According to the peer-reviewed American Journal of Respiratory and Critical Care Medicine, a recent study showed that stress during college final exams in students with mild asthma increased anxiety and depression and enhanced airway inflammation in response to antigens! Antigens are anything that causes the immune system to react, such as cat dander or ragweed pollen.

Viruses or colds

Viruses or colds may also be another way an asthma episode begins. Research completed at the University of Milan showed that two bacteria strains seem to be the culprits in asthma and the wheezing that accompanies it. The bacteria Mycoplasma pneumonia (Mpn) and Chlamydia pneumonia (Cpn) are present much more often in children with a history of asthma than those without it. Antibiotic therapy appeared to clear up symptoms of wheezing after three months. Viral infections have been a topic in the study for children's respiratory disease. It is thought that these viruses play a role in whether or not a child develops asthma! Respiratory syncytial virus (RSV) in children has been linked to the beginnings of asthma, with some speculation that there may be a genetic predisposition in some children to respond to this virus.

Bacteria and Fungus

In 2002, a study in a medical journal called <u>Chest</u> reported that 31 of 55 asthma patients studied had bacteria in the airways either Mycoplasma pneumoniaeor or another bacteria called Chlamydia (not the sexually transmitted type). At this time doctors admit that they do not have antibiotics that completely kill these organisms.

A leading bacterial/fungal theory comes to us from Germany. Dr. Gunther Enderlin studied the invasion of the host (our body) by a pathogenic factor or by our own internal mutation of the bacterium or fungus that we all may be carrying around. The internal workings of cellular function are affected by such an invasion leading to an anaerobic (without oxygen) respiration and congestion at the most basic level. Anaerobic respiration and congestion further spread into the internal milieu, which is a name given to all of the internal fluids of our internal environment. Once this corruption becomes widespread, the shift in the internal milieu will eventually affect our organs (our lungs for example) and lead to further accumulation of toxins that saturate the immune system with invaders to be fought. This proliferation of microorganisms can further be exacerbated by our lifestyle choices, especially stress. Stress on the body can also mean diet, water purity, and living environment.

In this world of the microbiological, another allergen factor is fungi. Since humans have altered the chemical environment internally (our bodes) and externally (our planet) more in the last 70 years than ever before in the history of our existence, it is no wonder that many of these microbes have mutated as well in order to survive. To illustrate, there are about 70,000 described species of fungi presently known (about 5%) living in a presumed world of about 1.5 million different species (95% unknown)! Fungi include all yeasts, mushrooms, mildew and molds. Fungi are the world's decomposers (like your compost heap in back of your garden) on a microscopic and macroscopic level. They live happily off of decaying tissue (parasitically) or off dying tissue (saprophytically). Fungi, according to Dr. Enderlin, are a higher form of pathology above virus and bacteria in complexity. In humans the existence of fungus is commonplace. They usually exist peacefully without causing harm.

However, when the body's milieu becomes out of balance (Yin and Yang) the fungi will multiply and begin to degrade the host (us), all the while producing toxins of their own! Candida, for example will produce about 75 of these canditoxons. While total elimination of these toxins is contraindicated and not advised, the process of bringing the body back to balance is. All processes in nature have "clean up" crews, from the vultures to the fungi. When this natural process becomes so disturbed by either over production or underproduction that the internal milieu supports rapid fungal growth and possibly other microbes, we lose the balance required by nature to be healthy. External factors such as diet, lifestyle and attitude can alter internal ecology such as immune function, microcirculation, microflora and, ultimately, the pH of the body. We will explain pH later in detail in Chap 5. Mycoplasma infection (the body's milieu becoming out of balance) has been a cofactor in AIDS, chronic fatigue, arthritis, respiratory infection, and urethritis. Further research on microbes has shown that *Helicobactor pylori* can lead to peptic and duodenal ulcers and some cancers and *Chlamydia pneumonia* to heart attacks and strokes.

Each asthma case is unique and deserves individual attention to discover what is truly out of balance. This microscopic world sometimes is blamed for a whole host of diseases. Still, we have a hard time understanding why something so small can be so powerful. We only see the top layer of the carnage, when the immune system gets so overwhelmed that it begins to mount its defenses.

I am currently exploring how to combat the bacteria Mycoplasma pneumonia (Mpn) and Chlamydia pneumonia (Cpn) using isopathic and pleomorphic type therapies combined with Chinese herbals and Qigong exercises.

The Trigger

The common link between these precursors is that they persuade the immune system to begin an inflammatory response. The body believes it is under attack by allergens, irritants, a cold or virus. The body mounts a counter offensive, which, unfortunately, means airway constriction for us and the forming of excess mucous.

One of the things that I notice is that you can actually feel when an apartment, house, school or any living area has the propensity for giving you an allergically induced asthma attack. We have to be aware of these trigger mechanisms as a means of self-defense. How is it possible to do this? Many times you can smell such things as damp and mold; the nose will begin to itch, the throat will begin to constrict or a contact allergy on the skin will start to bubble underneath. These are all warning signals to get out of that situation, otherwise the body is going to be under attack.

If you have this disease, it is good to know precisely what and how the body is doing especially if you are going to do your own research or explain it to your children in an accurate way. Children can take the truth. I know I wanted to hear it. When I was young, I always though my body was just "stupid" and deficient and that was why I was not like other kids. I needed to know the truth, that my body just "was a little more efficient and sensitive" than those of other kids. My body reacted to protect me, not to punish me.

Somewhere, there may be another child who thinks the way I thought. I hope that child reads this book and can straighten out this misunderstanding before the child feels negatively about him or herself.

CHAPTER 3

Anatomy 101, The Basic Stuff

Breathing, often taken for granted, does many wondrous things automatically (aside from keeping us alive). In a given day, the average person takes 20,000 breaths! Breathing normally allows us to have normal speech as well as to sigh and to laugh. Without our being consciously aware, breathing assists in the body's movement of blood and lymphatic flow. Breathing is like an internal massage that allows the spine to be mobile by the expansion of the rib cage and the musculature below (later I will show you how to breathe with your lower back area!) The normal exchange of the gases of oxygen and carbon dioxide facilitated by the breathing process allows the brain as well as all the organs, including the organs of digestion, and the tissue responses of the body to stay stabilized and operating at peak performance. We will divide this anatomy chapter into three subchapters of importance to asthma and allergies: the lungs, the brain and the skin.

The Lungs

The lungs transport oxygen to the rest of the body with the help of the heart, blood vessels and blood, also called the circulatory system. The lungs themselves have an immense capillary network that forms the surface tissue. The area of the lungs that does "breathing" is not physically attached to the rest of the body. You may have heard of the "lung sacs," which is a double walled sac separated by a thin space filled with fluid. One wall of the sac attaches to the outside of the lung itself, and the outer layer of the sac attaches to the chest cavity. This is like two panes of glass stuck together by water; you can slide them against each other, but you have a tough time pulling them apart.

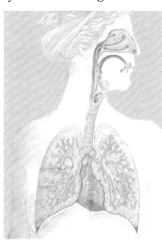

Lungs and complete airway

Air Passages: Anatomy 101, The Basic Stuff

The breathing cycle begins with the nose and mouth. I always envisioned this system of airflow by taking the visual part of a tree with all its branches and inverting it. The trunk of the tree is the nose, where the air is warmed, filtered by nose hairs and humidified. Next, the air travels down to the pharynx, where the pathways for food and air cross. The opening for air here is called the glottis, which extends to the Adam's apple or larynx. This is where your voice box which allows you to talk and sing is located. We are still envisioning the trunk of the tree so far. Next comes the trachea, or what we call the windpipe.

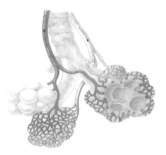

Enlarged view of aveoli airsacs

The trachea (windpipe) now branches out into two pathways called the bronchus. The left and right main bronchus leads to each lung on either side of the sternum or where the tree becomes the two main branches. It is interesting to note that the right and left main bronchus are not uniform; the left main bronchus is longer than the right. The right bronchus has three distinct "branches," or lobes, and the left has two. These branches break down even more minutely into bronchi and bronchioles or smaller and smaller versions of branches (actually to me they look like tentacles from an octopus) that give way to the alveolar sacs that remind me of a clump of fish eggs attached to each other. Ingeniously designed, the lymphatic system does have access to the bronchi and bronchioles, but not the alveoli themselves, further protecting the delicate alveoli from infection.

Breathing is usually controlled by the autonomic (I always think of "automatic") nervous system, of which there are two branches. One is the sympathetic, which is the part of the nervous system that is responsible for increase in heart rate, respiration and pulse.

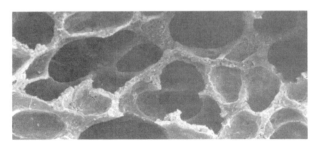

Enlarged view of aveoli airsacs

Some call this the fight or flight response. If this response is used in a physical event such as running from danger that is fine, but if it is in response to being yelled at by your boss that is a whole other matter. This state of overstimulation can lead to increased anxiety, hyperventilation or panic attacks. In fact, many times panic attacks are the result of an inaccurate breathing technique called hyperventilation.

The parasympathetic system offers the opposite effect. It calms and pacifies the whole organism. The parasympathetic system is what we need to control chronic stress. I will be working with you in developing and creating tools to control this system later in the book. The "higher" centers of the brain used when we think, sing, speak, or even when we are startled, can override the primitive brainstem that normally regulates breathing.

The Brain

The three-pound brain is a living dynamic ecosystem the physiology of which is still in the process of being mapped and deciphered. When stimulated properly, it can physically regenerate and adapt itself to a host of injuries. There are three divisions of the brain: 1)the brain stem, 2)the cerebellum and 3)the cerebrum. According to researcher Dr. Paul MacLean of the National Institutes of Health they have evolved into three distinct but interrelated subregions.

The Brain Stem or the Reptilian Brain

The brain stem was the first part of the brain to evolve - not only in the womb, but in the very first animals to walk the earth. Lizards had only this piece of the brain, hence the name "reptilian brain." The brain stem sits on top of the spinal column in a very protected area of the skull. This is for good reason, as the brain stem controls breathing, sleeping and waking, swallowing, and other automatic functions that go on even if you are knocked unconscious, like heartbeat. It relies on the senses for information, but no emotional feeling or logical deductive reasoning.

The Cerebellum or Limbic Brain

The limbic brain is sometimes called the mammalian brain or the emotional brain. Here is where the brain starts to really operate the coordination of your muscles, allowing you to move, to speak, to care for your child, to play and to exhibit empathy and caring. This is the part of the brain that athletes train to do complex movements like martial arts or dance.

The Limbic system is further divided into three areas, and terms you may have heard before Hippocampus, Amygdala and Cingulate Gyrus. The Hippocampus holds things like ideas or concepts you learn in college or this book's information and decides if they are novel or ordinary. The Amygdala holds emotional memories and decides how much importance or weight each event carries and how to react emotionally to each of these events. The Hypothalamus (the main control center for the autonomic nervous system) controls hunger, thirst, sexual function and body temperature; it decides how much adrenaline to send out during fight, fright or flight and works in conjunction with the Amygdala, the Hippocampus and the Neocortex (site of higher brain function) in deciding what priority an event has to the body. The Hypothalamus relay system then goes to the Pituitary gland and then out to the rest of the body (see chart next page).

The cingulate gyrus relays information between the emotional world of the limbic system and the decision-making process of the frontal lobe. Hyperactivity in this region may contribute to Tourette's syndrome; characterized by increased movement such as muscular and vocal tics, facial grimacing, pacing, twirling, coughing, sniffing, and grunting. Very recent research indicates the front portion of cingulate gyrus is involved in the emotional reaction to painful and other aversive events.

The limbic area is the part of the brain that psychiatrists Thomas Lewis, Fari Amini, and Richard Lannon state is increasingly important for the emotion we call love. In addition, the limbic connection between mammals, like the parent child bond or even common social contact, physiologically shapes and changes our evolving limbic brain. Interestingly enough, this is accomplished by what these scientists call resonance, or what I like to call vibration.

The Cerebrum or Neocortex

The Cerebrum is the largest part of the brain and the one that we "think" of when we refer to the brain. The left (logical and analytical thought) and right (face recognition, music, and creativity) brain halves are joined and together form a sphere that is covered by a thin layer called the neocortex. This two millimeter thick film is the part of the body that defines "you" in your consciousness awareness and it has been referred to as the "gray matter". From here, we divide the cerebrum into four areas or lobes: the frontal lobe (abstract problem solving); the paretial lobe sitting behind the frontal lobe (information processing from your sensory input); the occipital lobe sitting at the base of the brain (dedicated to vision) and the temporal lobe on the sides of the brain (memory, hearing and language).

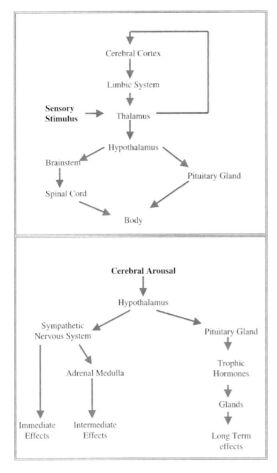

The linking mechanism between the two higher centers of the brain, the Limbic system and the Cerebral Cortex, is the reticular activating system (RAS). This RAS system works like a toggle switch that is diametrically thrown when we are emotionally pumped or when we relax. Arousal of any sort such as the fight, fright, or flight mechanism, triggers the RAS to shut down the cerebral cortex, the area that allows us to learn, and we resort to our "training." Conversely, if the Limbic system is switched off by the RAS, then relaxation takes place and so does creativity, as the higher center of the cerebral cortex take command.

I will use many of these terms later in the book when I discuss theories about asthma and explain meditation and Chinese Medicine. From what we understand currently, there are two major Western theories to explain asthma, the Beta Blocker theory and the Immune system response.

Beta Blocker Theory

This theory looks at how the nervous system affects the respiratory system. Internally, the nervous system and the immune system work with the respiratory system.

The central nervous system (brain, spinal cord, and connecting nerves) works like a messenger service with the brain acting as the dispatcher, the nerves as the actual messenger, and the spinal column as the pathway or highway to facilitate communication.

There are two divisions of the nervous system: the Autonomic Nervous System (ANS), which controls the involuntary processes, those without the need for conscious thought (like heart rate, blood pressure, food digestion, etc.) and the Central Nervous System (CNS).

We now know that the CNS, especially the cerebral cortex, hypothalamus, and the medulla oblongata, regulates the ANS. The two divisions are still taught in medical schools as two separate systems for convenience of study, not necessarily for accuracy in operation.

Within the Autonomic Nervous System there are two subdivisions: the sympathetic and the parasympathetic systems. The sympathetic system prepares the body for "Fight, Fright or Flight" quickens the heart rate, relaxes bronchial tubes, quickens breathing, dilates blood vessels and the pupils, releases epinephrine or adrenaline, and a host of other responses. These are the very same responses we have in stressful situations, whether they are real or imagined. As we understand these systems further, we will begin to understand how the mind can play an important role in controlling these body functions augmenting the mind and mind-tools (meditation) to new levels of healing.

The parasympathetic system actually acts in the opposite way; it counters the effects of the sympathetic system. The parasympathetic system uses a neurotransmitter called acetylcholine and is actually more in control during sleep. The body has its own set of checks and balances and works perfectly to balance the opening and narrowing of the bronchial tubes in a normal pair of lungs. In the asthmatic lung, however, this delicate control system is tipped toward the parasympathetic system and constriction happens. Although the parasympathetic system is heavily involved, it is not believed at this time to be the main culprit in asthma attacks.

Just like a trucking company, the nerves communicate by having the trucks carrying the messengers (the neurotransmitters) to the docks or receiving ends (the receptors). Now let us delve a little deeper into the actual neurotransmitters, the epinephrine and the acetylcholine. Each of these chemical messengers is only one of many actual neurotransmitters the nerves use to communicate with each other.

The docks or receptors control all body functions and subdivide into Alpha, Beta1, and Beta2 type receptors. Alpha-receptors manage to raise heart rate, tighten bronchial tubes and increase mucous production.

Beta1 receptors act on the heart muscle itself; they raise blood pressure, relax bronchial muscles, and decrease mucous secretion. Some research indicates that people with asthma may have abnormal beta-receptors. Their neurotransmitters (trucks) are blocked from reaching their destination: the receptors (the docks). This block is not normal to the body; it throws the parasympathetic system into a tizzy and causes the nerves to overreact and constrict bronchial tubes.

Beta2 receptors are common in the airway muscles themselves. Most of the beta-agonists inhalators (like Albuterol) work on the Beta2 receptors in the lungs but can also speed up the heart rate by affecting the Beta1 receptors at the same time.

Immune System Response

The immune system is unique in the fact that it is a learning organism. The immune system recognizes, like an elite squadron of commandos, what is foreign and domestic to the body. It actively seeks out and destroys the foreign invaders, which are typically proteins. What is even more amazing is that it is relentless in its attack on foreigners. It will never quit or retreat once in battle with a foreign invader. It's like Bruce Lee, Arnold Schwarzenegger as the Terminator, and Rocky morphing together, all coming to fight on your side.

The main players here are the thymus gland located in your lower neck, the lymphatic system, and the bone marrow which produces the two types of blood cells: red and white. Red blood cells transport oxygen from the lung tissue to the body via a vast network of arteries and arterioles. The white blood cells use the same transportation pathways to defend the body against infection. Lymphocytes are a type of white blood cell. Lymphocytes are further broken down to B (bone) cells and T (thymus) cells. Bone marrow produces about a billion white blood cells a day! B cells manufacture antibodies (an immunoglobulin molecule) that pair with a specific antigen (the invader). These antibodies then identify the antigen as the enemy so the immune system response can seek and destroy the antigen. The white blood cells release a special cell called a T cell. B cells, the radio operator in the army, communicate with the T cells.

Antibodies also record the type of invader so that the next time it comes into the body, the response time to destroy it is much faster. When a T cell meets its mortal enemy, the antigen, it begins to replicate itself and destroy the invader. The T cells release a substance called cytokines that actually do the destroying of the invader. The cytokines, like a general in charge, regulate the intensity and duration of the immune response to the antigen. You may have heard of interferon and interleukin, which are actually cytokines.

Immunoglobulin E

Immunoglobulin E (IgE) is a type of antibody that supposedly evolved in our ancestors to ward off parasites, and is still released in our bodies today by B cells. Unfortunately, some people produce far more than they ever need (up to 20 times what they could ever use). This means that your body overreacts to common substances (allergens) that produce asthma. Each allergen produces a different IgE antibody. These IgE antibodies attach themselves to cells in the nose, airways, and skin and throughout the body. These cells are called mast cells.

Mast Cells

Mast cells reside in the lungs and the intestines and are critical to asthma suffers. Mast cells are highly attracted to IgE but are also sensitive to food antigens. How long and how rough your asthma attack is depends on how well the IgE and the mast cells play together along with histamine and arachidonic acid. Inside the mast cell is a chemical called histamine. Histamine, secreted by mast cells, releases strong chemicals into the surrounding tissue giving rise to reddening and swelling of the tissue including the bronchioles. Hives, sneezing, runny nose, mucous production, wheezing and coughing are some of the by-products of activation. Antihistamines (Benadryl) are the common relief mechanism generally used to deal with this reaction.

Arachidonic acid is derived from linoleic acid, an essential omega-6 fatty acid, is found in overabundance in modern diets (vegetable oils). Arachidonic acid is than converted to eicosanoids (an inflammation causing compound) and joins with a protein called cytokines. These cytokines have names like C-reactive protein, which has a blood test of the same name, to measure inflammation in the artery walls.

Mast cells release another chemical called leukotrienes (derived from arachidonic acid mentioned earlier), which cause prolonged constriction of the airway muscles.

Another chemical created by the body, eosinophils, is believed to increase airway sensitivity and inflammation.

When I was growing up in the sixties, asthma was thought of as restrictive airway disease. In other words, the asthmatic patient could not get enough air into the lungs because of the constriction and mucous.

Other Current Theories

Now, we know that asthma is not about getting enough air. Asthma is about getting the correct balance of oxygen to carbon dioxide in a balanced Yin and Yang state (see chapter 12). You see in one scenario, the stale, used air actually is trapped inside the lungs and the body cannot dispense it through normal means. This old stale air is full of carbon dioxide, which is poisonous to the body. This gas is a by-product of normal respiration, but when the balance tips through inflammation, which leads to congestion and mucous, too much of this gas builds up. Since the airways are filled with old air, there is no room for fresh oxygenated air to enter.

Another theory of how asthma begins involves high levels of the hormone estrogen and the mother. Scientists established a link between the age a mother started menstruating and whether their child had allergies or not. They found that mothers who started menstruating early, before the age of fifteen, had conditions in the womb that might set the stage for allergies in the child and had children with a greater prevalence of allergies.

There are also other theories, for example that we are "too clean" during our early development. Researchers at Columbia University hypothesized that if the immune system is only exposed to hygienic, sterile environments and not allowed to acclimate itself to various allergens in infancy that the immune system overreacts later in life and contributes to the hyperactivity of asthma attacks. Combine this with the huge volume of chemical products we use today that are antibacterial and antimicrobial. These products kill germs and temporarily sanitize, but on the other hand expose us to chemicals not found in nature. Therefore, the very cleaners designed to "help us" are foreign themselves to the body and our immune system.

There is also the theory that we use emergency inhalators to frequently, instead of being selective in our conditions of inhaler use and environments. It is much more convenient to take a puff from an inhalator than to avoid the food we love, to warm up adequately before exercise or avoid the room with the cigarette smoke. Frequent and overuse of these emergency inhalators can lead to their ineffectiveness and compound the cycle of asthma attack/inhalator use further.

The Skin

Let us analyze the skin a little bit. Skin is actually the largest organ of the body; it encompasses 22 square feet and weighs around 9 pounds on an average man. This semipermeable membrane is actually composed of two layers, the outer thinner part called the epidermis and the thicker tissue beneath called the dermis. The epidermis is the part that many times becomes damaged and opens due to scratching from allergic irritation, rashes and small pimple-like structures. Under the dermis is the subcutaneous layer sometimes called the superficial fascia and contains adipose tissue or fat.

The skin is an extension of our nervous system and therefore can reflect our physiological and emotional states. Diseases from the internal organs can manifest themselves on the skin, such as jaundice from the liver and paleness from blood anemia.

Skin Inflammation & Allergic Itching

I always thought of skin inflammation in a negative way, but as I understand more, it is quite the normal response for the body to go through. In fact, it is the body's way to begin healing itself. The redness, swelling, heat and, sometimes, pain, are evidence that the immune system is in operating order and doing its job. The problem begins if this is the constant state of affairs.

The problem is how to contend with the misery of the redness and itching, especially at night when your mental defense of "don't scratch" is turned off.

If you itch because of allergies: make sure you keep your nails short to keep yourself from scratching at night and opening up your skin. Make your sleeping quarters a cool and dry place free from dust, mold, mildew and dust mites. In other words, reduce the humidity and the temperature in the room substantially from the rest of the house by running either a dehumidifier or air conditioner. Germs and molds have a much harder time living in a cool dry place than a moist warm one. Air conditioners and dehumidifiers need to be cleaned frequently to prevent bacteria from forming and then being blown around the room.

Change your bed sheets frequently and often, at least every three days during periods of exacerbation of skin flare-ups. When your skin is healing and flaking off at a higher than normal rate dust mites can build up quickly in the very sheets you lie in.

EPA studies have shown that our homes are up to 200% more polluted than the outdoor environment. In newer homes (or newly remodeled homes) this is due in part to the off-gassing of building materials like plywood, chemical paints and varnishes, plastic piping, and even the fibers and dyes used in your carpets, upholstery and window treatments. Keeping the windows closed and the indoor air recirculating is trapping all this pollution in your home. In dealing with these chemical stresses your immune system is so busy it doesn't have the energy or ability to fight off the cold or the flu.

Another major pollutant in our homes is the chemicals we use to clean our floors, bathrooms, dishes and clothes. Most of the ingredients in those chemical cleaners are not good for your health, yet we use them constantly and fill our immediate surroundings with them.

A few simple changes can be made that can make an instant impact, especially if someone in your home suffers from allergies or other skin irritations. Dust mites are the terrible little creatures that eat dust (most dust particles are flakes of our own skin!), and these mites LOVE to live in your bed. While this is good for the mites as they get an ample amount of food there, their excrement causes allergies and skin irritations. Normal detergents may add chemicals to your sheets and bedclothes, and may not necessarily kill the mites. A cup of Borax (20 Mule Team) in each wash load will kill any mites in the bedding and will discourage others from living in this fabric. Try using a more natural washing powder like Arm and Hammer, to reduce further irritations. Using 100 percent cotton bedding with natural dyes will reduce chemical stress further.

Wash your hands as often as you can remember and every time you remember. This reduces contact allergies from invading the body and keeps you from spreading germs and infection to other parts of your body, like your eyes. If you have dry skin and skin allergies, make sure that you use a hand cream to replenish the natural oils you just washed off.

Cotton and silk clothing seem to be the most comfortable on the skin and allow it to breathe. Many other types of clothing like wool seem to irritate, and may actually cause an allergic reaction. Another thing to remember is to have clothing that "breathes" for normal perspiration and cooling of your body.

Many people are sensitive to the metal nickel. Nickel is used in dental fillings and in the backs of earrings and other jewelry. Nickel allergy is one of the most common contact allergies for women. If your child has allergies, you may want to think twice about getting their ears pierced.

If you know you are allergic to ragweed, you may not know that some of your favorite foods may have the same protein that causes you to itch. Watermelon, cantaloupes, honeydew, cucumbers, and zucchini all have the same protein according, to the Allergy Research Laboratory of Detroit's Henry Ford Hospital.

Be aware of sulfites. Sulfites are used everywhere in our attempt to produce, pack, ship and store food faster and longer than ever before. The FDA has banned sulfites in supermarket produce or in your favorite restaurants because they have lead to fatalities over the years. Sulfites release sulfur dioxide gas as we chew and drink. If you have asthma or allergies to sulfites, be aware that by chewing, eating or drinking slowly you can have a greater awareness of the warning signs of an attack. Flushing, itching, coughing, wheezing, or a warm feeling all can be signals that your body is trying to tell you something. The FDA ban does not apply to potatoes and their products, frozen and canned vegetables or wine and beer.

I personally like to use Pycnogenol crème or Retinol and Green Tea crème from Derm-E. I like the way these crèmes feel on my skin and they do not build up as much residue on the skin surface which later can trap dirt and cause bacteria to grow. These trapped bacteria will further exacerbate the itching process.

Aloe Vera is a wonderful tonic to soothe and moisturize irritated skin. I have used it successfully to calm my irritated skin and calm the itch of an allergic reaction. There are many aloe products on the market and I think I have tried them all. In my consumer watchdog role, I have found certain products that add many other ingredients to their aloe typically lose the effectiveness of the aloe. Find one that is pure aloe and stick with it. I have found that Banana Boat Aloe Vera is the most comfortable on my skin, although there can be coloring added.

I have added, experimented and used other products in combination with the aloe and some work better than the others. When I am extremely itchy, Benadryl lotion mixed with the aloe applied after wiping the area clean seems to work well. I will also mix in cortisone creme, as the ointment version seems to clog my pores more.

Speaking of cleaning the skin, I have found that people with allergies that are severe enough to break out the epidermal layer usually have a host of other problems, like dry skin. Having dry skin means that a moisturizer is needed, but also one that does not clog the skin pores. The clogged pores can lead to more itching and irritation, especially in hot and/or humid weather. The best product I have found is called AmLactin. It is the same formula as a prescription named ProLactin, but AmLactin can be bought over the counter; and, at least at the writing of this book, is available for 1/3 of the cost. I understand that there is a court case going on about this and we will have to see what happens as the drug companies do battle. Mix the Amlactin (1 part) with Aloe Vera (3 parts) for a silky moisturizing lotion.

Tea tree crème is a wonderful soothent for red itchy skin. Oil from the Tea Tree (Melaleuca Alternifolia) has been used for centuries as an anesthetic, and antibacterial, antifungal agent. I typically mix it with Aloe again to make a silky mixture. I have also found that avocado creme is non-clogging and moisturizing as well, especially on the face.

Cleaning the skin with alcohol or peroxide sometimes helps to cut the itch. I have found that itching sometimes is caused by a combination of sweat, dirt, creams, and lotion residue built up over time. Typically soap and water do not cut through this layer of scum on the skin and therefore the skin begins to "suffocate" and itch. Alcohol, peroxide or other commercial skin-cleansers appear to be needed lifestyle maintenance for keeping the skin free of scum buildup. This is especially true during the summer months when there is more pollen in the air that lies on the skin (contact allergies). The propensity to sweat more makes the mixture viscous. You may also try witch hazel as a cleanser on the skin.

I am an authority on contact allergies from experience. Everything from pine tree pollen to dog hair to various commercial soaps seemed to irritate my skin and cause itch. I found the faster I could clean off the allergen lying on my skin, the more control I would have from itching and the breaking open of my skin from scratching. I used to carry a little bottle filled with the following formula and some cotton balls in my jacket, as I never knew what I would be getting into.

The homemade formula I invented is isopropyl alcohol (about 55%), baking soda, fresh lemon juice, and water. You will have to adjust the baking soda thickness to your liking with water. I usually do this before adding the alcohol and lemon. Use a loofa sponge to apply and rub gently. I find that this formula works well when I am irritated from contact allergies. You can make enough of a quantity to store and use again, as there is nothing to break down. Make sure you seal it well with a tight lid in your designated container, as the alcohol will evaporate. Try a small area first to see if this formula agrees with you, as our sensitivities are all different.

Make sure you moisturize your skin with fresh aloe vera and Alpha Lipoic Acid, as the above formula will dry your skin. Derma-E makes a very nice DMAE, Alpha Lipoic Acid and C-Ester creme that feels good on my skin, is not greasy and hydrates the skin tissue.

CHAPTER 4
The Theory of Hyperoxigenation

We have Dr. Otto Warbug of Germany to thank for the theory of hyperoxigenation. Dr. Warbug won the Nobel Prize for medicine in 1931 for proving that cancer is anaerobic; it cannot reproduce or even survive in a high oxygen environment. Furthering this research about oxygen was Dr. Manfred von Ardenne who was Dr. Warbug's student. Until his death in 1997, Dr. von Ardenne, an electron physicist, worked on his theory of respiratory psychophysiology. He called this research Oxygen Multistep Therapy.

The air we breathe is comprised of several different chemicals. Oxygen, which surprisingly only comprises about 21% of our atmosphere, is what we are most concerned with. Oxygen is 90% of the weight of water. If we think about our body in weight; our body is 75% water. Therefore, with a little math: the body is 63% oxygen! Think of the implications of that. Every cell in our body needs oxygen to survive, but the quantity we need to keep our cells happy may be compromised.

The quality of air that we breathe is another question. Certainly, we can tell a comparative difference in how the air feels when we are in Los Angeles or Beijing, China to the freshness of Yosemite National Park or on a ranch in Montana. Extreme examples, I know, but they illustrate a point of air quality variance that we may never consider a factor in our health. In fact, oxygen content in the air we breathe may drop as much as 10% in the city. [1]

Receiving enough of the pure elements of air into our bodies and expelling the contaminated and used elements is the way nature intended us to function. In our modern society, we often do not physically work hard enough to breathe deeply to use the full volume or capacity of our lungs. This is especially true as we age. How many times do 40 or 50 year-olds run till they are out of breath and gasping as they did when they were children? We now call physical exertion exercise, but originally it was called survival and work. Additionally, more tasks were completed outside in fresh, circulating air than are today.

Air Passages: The Theory of Hyperoxigenation

Modern office buildings, homes and schools are more airtight and energy efficient than ever. This leads to another potential problem in off-gassing, lack of circulation of carbon dioxide out of the building and such issues as radon gas, carbon monoxide etc. All of these gases are invisible and most are undetectable by the nose. Exposure to these gases is inevitable, especially in the newest of homes.

The more concrete we pour and the more trees we cut down the worse off we are in air quality. Homeostasis and a balance of Yin / Yang applies here. The tree is actually a living HEPA filtering plant that removes toxins from the air and spews back pure oxygen. The less you are around these marvelous wonders of nature, the more *your* body becomes the filtering plant of toxins (something it is not designed to do).

Combining the lack of air quality with our lack of movement in the United States at near epidemic levels, and we have the makings of a national health problem. Fifty-five percent of all Americans are overweight or obese. This is even more true for the asthmatic than the average person. The asthmatic is many times afraid to be active because of risk of asthma attack!

Obviously, the body needs oxygen, but the body does not really have an "oxygen sensor." What the body does have is sensitivity to the pH level. When we take in a breath of air it is transported to our bloodstream via the red blood cells containing hemoglobin. When cellular respiration or work uses the oxygen, carbon dioxide and water are the by-products. When carbon dioxide mixes with water it forms carbonic acid and begins to drop the pH level of the body. A relay system picks this up and sends the message to the part of the brain called the brainstem (actually the medulla and the pons). This is the primitive part of the brain, mentioned earlier called the reptilian brain. Through a series of chemical reactions, the body sends messages to increase oxygen intake to alkalize the blood to bring the pH level back to balance again.

Whew! All of that goes on in seconds within the body. Talk about a workhorse. When the pH level falls or becomes acidic from too much carbon dioxide, the autonomic nervous system kicks in and takes control again to regulate and increase the amount of oxygen provided to the cells.

Air Passages: The Theory of Hyperoxigenation

Breathing correctly affects every single tissue in your body, your metabolism, heart rate and its function, and the body's ability to control its own pH level (acid to base ratio) [2]. PH level is something you may have heard about - it is vital to existence. Waste disposal from tissues themselves (cellular metabolism), metabolic rate (dictated by activity level, and food nutrients) and oxygen intake (whether through activity level or breathing technique) all affect the body's pH level. If the body's pH level does not remain at a constant 7.3 to 7.4, especially in blood (slightly alkaline), your life can be in danger. Water has a pH level of 7.0 (neutral).

All of us have learned in high school biology class that we expel carbon dioxide as a waste gas from our lungs. What we may not understand is that the correct amount of carbon dioxide must be expelled. This is another example of the world existing in a Yin/Yang balance that cannot be interrupted. While it is a toxic gas, the body must have a certain amount of carbon dioxide gas within the lungs to maintain homeostasis. The body must be balanced in the correct ratio of gases for correct pH level as well as for healthy optimal breathing. In fact, according to some proponents of the Konstantin Buteyko method, the exchange ratio should be about 6 percent CO_2 to 2 percent oxygen.

Excessive exhalation (lots of sighs) or hyperventilation as part of a usual breathing pattern can lead to increased respiration. Perceived pain, such as receiving a shot at the dentist, or worrying or dreading taking a test, can cause increased respiration. This excess purging of CO_2, or carbon dioxide, moves the pH scale toward an alkaline state. By breathing too little or not deeply enough, the pH drops into the acidic range because more carbon dioxide is retained. For example, we naturally produce more carbon dioxide when we exercise, but the body in its wisdom also purges more CO_2 by increased respiration and deeper breathing mechanics. However, things like excessive muscle contraction from stress (your tense neck and shoulders) can produce more carbon dioxide without the means of dispensing the excess evenly. If the expected fight or flight muscle activity is not produced in an expected period of time, the body will have a crisis on its hands. The human being is almost a perfect creation, except when one's own mind interrupts the natural cycles of breathing and pH levels. It seems that there is this one subroutine in the computer program that can throw the entire system out of whack and that monkey wrench is the mind itself.

What I am about to say next may really throw everything we have been taught about asthma on its ear. Asthmatics breathe differently than other people. No news there, but the ratio of inhale to exhale to pause between each cycle is what is altered! What I have learned through trial and error and studying Eastern breathing methods is that we breathe too fast and do not pause between our breaths. We never allow our body to settle with what oxygen we have taken in, which allows the body to build up enough carbon dioxide in the alveoli of the lungs to bring the body to homeostasis (balance).

Some asthmatics have a tendency to overbreathe or breathe too fast in their day-to-day breathing. When this happens we lose too much carbon dioxide and the blood pH changes so that the blood cannot actively release its reserves of oxygen to the cells that so desperately need it. Although there is plenty of oxygen being taken in, the body is out of pH balance; therefore, the amount of oxygen utilization is minimal at best. This can be one cause of, or exacerbate, an asthma attack.

I conduct stress seminars all over the country. One of my first experiments with the audience is to see how they have conditioned themselves to:

      1. Breathe with the intercostal muscle (ribs or chest)

      2. Breathe with the diaphragm or stomach.

The results always astound me. Almost two thirds of the audience breathes with their chest (intercostals), with a few breathing with both intercostals and the full diaphragm. Less than one fourth actually breathe with their full diaphragm capacity! From the empirical evidence I have gathered so far, 75% of Americans breathe inefficiently!

Asthmatics do have a tendency to be very tight in their breathing the result of unconscious muscular contraction of their neck and chest. Day-to-day stress and fear of the asthma attack itself makes asthmatics "hold" their bodies in a very rigid type of physiology. As we do when we know something is going to hurt, we "brace ourselves" or tense our muscles for the pain/attack that is about to come. I say this out of experience, and I am not saying that this holding pattern is the cause of asthma, just one of the contributing factors to its exacerbation.

Air Passages: The Theory of Hyperoxigenation

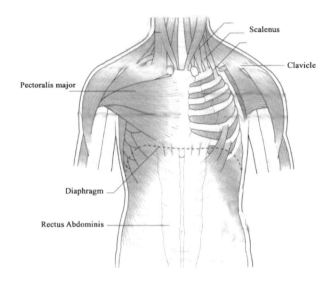

When I look at severe asthmatics, I notice a radical difference in their posture. The over-contraction of certain muscles and the over-stretching of others gives the posture a rounded look. Classically, as a result several muscle groups need to be stretched back to their original position and others have to be strengthened. The exercises I will outline for you in later chapters 7 and 14 will do precisely this. I am always learning new exercises, so don't feel that this is a complete list, but it will give you a nice starter package.

The muscles I see over-contracted (shortened) are the brachial plexus, the pectoralis minor and major, the scalenus, the upper trapezius (T1) and the levator scapulae. Conversely, I see weak rhomboids, serratus anterior, rectus abdominous, and lower and middle trapezius muscles (T3 T4). This causes change in the head posture and affects C1 and C2 vertebra. Many times I see in the clinic a further progression to Thoracic Outlet Syndrome, where pain then shoots down the arm into the hand. Sometimes people even think they have carpel tunnel because of this.

Learning to truly relax and take back control of the breathing system is what I have learned in saving my own life many times. Exercises, visualizations and breathing methods can be taught to asthmatics to support efficient breathing mechanisms. I will teach these to you in this book and give you everything you need to be proactive in your own health care and healing journey.

Three Regions of Breath

The three regions of breath in order of rest to exertion are: the full diaphragm (belly breathing), the chest (intercostals) and the clavicle area (the collarbones).

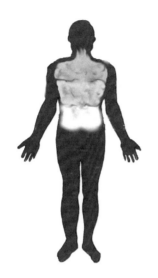

We only use the clavicle area during extreme exertion such as running a 100-yard dash for time. Notice when football players rush downfield for a touchdown what part of their anatomy is heaving at the goal line. Like the top of a teardrop, the lungs actually extend up toward the clavicles. This part of the lung is only used for oxygen exchange when every single alveoli is used for moving precious oxygen into the body's cells.

During our day-to-day activities, including moderate exercise, the clavicle is seldom used. An exception occurs in the person born with severe asthma, such as myself, who needs to use every millimeter of lung tissue to breathe in normal activities. An interesting side note: people like myself who have used clavicular breathing for extended periods of time, tend to develop increased muscle mass in the upper trapezius muscle (the neck muscle that looks like cantaloupes sitting on the shoulders of some wrestlers and bodybuilders).

As babies aligned with nature, we breathe with the lower belly or with a full diaphragm. Later, through nurture, the child learns to breathe shallowly when it is held against the chest of the mother (or father) and imitates the breathing pattern displayed by the adult. Since a baby learns first what is demonstrated to him or her, it is only natural to follow in the footsteps of its "teachers".

Pain is controlled through breathing techniques, specifically diaphragmatic breathing. An example is the Lamaze breathing techniques taught to pregnant women. Proper breathing not only aids asthmatics, but also can be used as a "natural cure" for such tension related pain as headaches and can unequivocally help with PMS, hot flashes, and insomnia.

The diaphragm is a muscle, just like your heart. Like your other muscles, you must use it or lose it. The only way to exercise the diaphragm is through the contraction process that occurs during abdominal breathing techniques. In reality, many people never fully use the diaphragm to its full capacity, an exception to this is someone trained in opera or music (wind instruments).

Another interesting fact about breathing with the diaphragm is that not only should your lower abdomen move (below your navel) but the lower back should also move! Back breathing has long been considered by the Asian martial arts as the center or root of a person's power. This little known fact has been a secret to martial arts masters for centuries. Unless the lower back moves on the inspiration of air, the diaphragm is not fully contracted and the tidal volume of air is not maximized.

Diaphragmatic breathing is more closely associated with relaxing and calming of the body whereas chest breathing is typically associated with activity or panic and fright. Notice someone who has just completed an exercise program at the gym, and see what part of his body is gulping in oxygen, or notice someone who is panic stricken and see where their breath originates.

Through muscular contraction the body allows the rib cage to expand and open the thoracic (chest) cavity of the body to provide more air to flow in through the trachea (windpipe). This muscular contraction does not necessarily contract the diaphragm, though. It is as if there are two different breathing apparatuses working here. In the breathing techniques I teach, I show people how to use all three anatomical parts plus how to move them in six directions to breathe more efficiently. We also show exercise to improve and develop these breathing mechanisms.

In addition to diaphragmatic breathing, there are six directions of breath that we need to think about in the inhale/exhale sequence. As you inhale, think about filling your torso with air from bottom to top, front to back and left and right. These six directions will give uniformity to your breathing sequence.

Train the body to use all 3 parts of breath in six directions!

In some respects, the body is so basic in terms of its design and optimal function. The body, its muscle, tendons and ligaments, the heart, lungs and blood, were meant to move and be used to their fullest potential. We are designed to stretch and bend and climb like an active 5-year-old. I believe we lose so much of this ability at a younger age now, more than at any other time in our history.

In my karate classes, I see young boys and girls so limited and tight in their movements I wonder how they are going to get by in adulthood without a back problem or a shoulder problem. I can see lower back problems and shoulder problems already starting to materialize at their young ages. Shoulder and chest flexibility, hamstring tightness, lack of abdominal strength, weak hands and wrists, limited range in squatting down are all indicators to me that they have not moved this way in some time.

The ability of the body to adapt and find balance within is fundamental to all training models. Every athlete, from high school player to Olympic contestant, understands the training process of pushing the body to adapt to greater and greater loads of stress. Whether this is through weight training, running, plyometrics, PNF stretching, or calisthenics, making the body perform to higher levels of skill is paramount for success. How we accomplish this is the subject that coaches, research scientists, and athletes themselves debate, refine, and experiment with continuously. Copious quantities of books, articles, seminars, news releases seminars and videotapes are produced every year on new and improved methods of optimal training techniques, performance through proper nutrition, supplements and herbals.

Have you ever thought of training the body for asthma?

Granted, these methods are crucial for improved training and performance. However, they neglect one very important ingredient that determines true success in athletics and all kinds of competition. That critical ingredient is proper breathing technique. Without proper oxygen/waste removal (pH balance) the body cannot process the ingested food it converts to fuel, nor power through tough workouts, let alone go up the stairs without gasping for air.

Moreover, another interesting point can be made that breathing can affect our mood and our emotions. In recent studies at Michigan, Pittsburgh and Stanford Universities, children who have inattention and hyperactivity disorders were shown to have as well sleep disturbed breathing and snoring. In fact, 39% of boys found to be hyperactive snored during sleep. Treating these sleep disturbances that cause hyperactivity could be treated with ancient breathing methods based on a Chinese exercise form called Qigong (discussed more in Chapter 14)

Every athlete needs to learn proper breathing to enhance performance. Every asthmatic, cancer patient, ADHD child, surgical patient, pain patient, and person with high blood pressure should be practicing breathing methods. In fact, there is not one person alive who could not benefit from breathing techniques. The secret is to get oxygen into the body to do the most good. Breathing technique is the catalyst that makes correct eating habits and exercise methods work to your chemical genetic potential.

In a recent study published in the New England Journal of Medicine, a few cents worth (about 3 cents) of oxygen administered after surgery can cut the risk of surgical infections in half and patients were less likely to be nauseated! The white blood cells (neutrophils) that are the body's army search and destroy the germs that cause infection. Scientists have proven that high oxygen levels in the body's tissues help to prevent infections. The doctors also hypothesized that oxygen therapy might be used to speed healing in burn and surgical patients.

The only problem is that too much oxygen in the body, especially artificially administered from an oxygen tank, can be harmful or even fatal to the body. A more natural way to oxygenate the body is through age-old QiGong breathing techniques or various yoga exercises proven for thousands of years. Through these methods the body uses its natural method of inspiration to pull atmospheric oxygen into the body and extract contaminants in a manner that it is accustomed to through thousands of years of biological adaptation. Anything that the body is not accustomed to can cause additional trauma to the body and raise the level of stress, the very thing that we are trying to eliminate.

Importing oxygen into the body is only half the issue; transporting the oxygen where it needs to be is the next step. To fully understanding how our asthma exercises work, we must now look at the job of the blood or more specifically, the hemoglobin.

Blood

We understand that oxygen is vital to life and blood is vital to life, but the interrelationship between the two is also critical to health. As the war rages on against terrorism, we speak of spilling blood or of innocent blood. Blood truly is the icon of life itself. We probably don't think of our blood often, except when we cut ourselves or we hear the Central Blood Bank plea for blood as their reserves run low. How often do we think of our own blood and its health? We probably think of it quite often if we are a cancer patient and are concerned about things like T-cells, and white blood cell count, or if we are an AIDS patient or a hemophiliac. Most of us, however, have little conscious thought about our blood's condition.

In Chinese Medicine, everything is about the blood, or Xue. The Chinese say that "Qi (our life force) is the commander of blood and blood is the mother of Qi". This statement speaks of the interrelationship between the Yin (blood) and Yang (Qi) in Chinese medicine theory where Yin is of Earth and Yang is of Heaven, or the tangible and the intangible. In Chinese medical diagnosis, we are concerned about blood stasis in trauma or disease, for instance. We also speak of injuring the blood through our emotions and our negative repetitive thoughts, which is very different, I admit, from the western science paradigm of blood and its functions. I have often thought about the similarities between Western medicine and Chinese or Tibetan medicine, and their preoccupation with the health of one's blood. For those of you who probably could care less about this, stay tuned because I will explain how this concept will help you to burn off those extra pounds so evilly placed around your midsection!

Blood is an amazing substance that is more of its own little ecosystem than we once thought. The pH of our body has an immense affect on our blood. If the pH of our blood becomes imbalanced ever so slightly, microbes can become pathogenic, enzymes can become destructive, and mineral assimilation can be thrown off, which leads to a state favoring yeast, viruses, bacteria and cancer.

To most of us, blood flows without our mental assistance or control. When we are healthy, it is in constant motion, forever orbiting the body in an endless loop like the Earth around the Sun. Regardless of how efficiently we can breath or how well we can digest our food, if it weren't for the blood acting as the trucking company traveling down a thousand mile highway system of arteries, arterioles and capillaries, we would soon die. In a healthy body, blood moves, sometimes slowly, but moves nonetheless, assisted by the contraction of muscles in the body (i.e. movement of the body). Movement of the body is imperative for the health of the blood, not only for the assistance it provides in moving the blood, but from the increased fresh supply of oxygen from our deeper breathing which facilitates our healing energies.

Long before Western physiology understood the Yin and Yang balance between blood and the lungs, the ancient Chinese realized the connection between breathing in oxygen and the health of the blood. Remember: on exhale, the lungs release carbon dioxide from the blood capillaries into the alveoli (air sacs); conversely, on inhale, fresh oxygen enters the alveoli and permeates the blood capillaries and then flows to the left side of the heart. Breathing exercises were studied and experimented with in order to study their effect on health, energy levels, and recuperation from illness. Therefore, blood and breathing became a very common treatment modality in ancient China.

Ironically, this vital substance called blood is under constant production as its shelf life is minimal. In an average day, 100 billion neutrophils (a type of white blood cell) are produced by an average adult, but what is more incredible is that this liquid is produced in a solid....the bone! The Chinese even have special exercise called Marrow Washing QiGong; that is used to build up the blood cell production. I use this form of exercise a lot with several of my cancer clients as well as people who are anemic. Both east and west recognize the importance of blood health, but have different methods of treating diseases of the blood.

Movement and deep breathing, regardless of its nature, is how the body was designed to function. It doesn't matter if you do pilates or yoga, run, or lift weights, the important factor is that you are moving your blood. Think of how you can move more and stop thinking of it as exercise! If you want to change how you look on the outside, change what will affect your health the most, your blood...... from the inside out.

Changing the blood means synergistically changing one's diet and incorporating correct exercise, meditation and breathing techniques. This is my personalized method of obtaining optimal health.

Now the tricky part is the correct combination of the triad, and knowing the correct hierarchy. I will give you a complete triad itinerary.

The body is an organism that is very adaptive in nature. This can work for us or against us. If you lie on the couch and eat bonbons all day long, that is what your body will adapt to as its comfort zone. May God help you if you ever do any very physical activity for very long because you will pay dearly with aching muscles and/or by pulling or popping something out of joint.

On the other hand, if you train the body to become efficient in its ability to squeeze oxygen out of every morsel of atmosphere you give it, then that is what your body will become. Think of how people have to adapt to high altitudes. Several thousand feet can make a dramatic difference in your ability to obtain oxygen, but given several days or weeks, just about everyone can adapt.

THE BASIC PREMISE IS THIS: YOU NEED TO CREATE A SLIGHT DEFICIT IN AVAILABILITY OF OXYGEN TO THE CELLS.

Once this demand or deficit has been accomplished, my specialized breathing therapies "reload" the cells with fresh clean oxygen plus a little more. The body, being conservative in nature, will want a reserve tank of oxygen on board for the next activity and will adapt to breathe more efficiently.

During this period of oxygen reloading, the body also reduces its stress, quiets the pulse, reduces blood pressure and begins to heal as when you sleep while you are sick. This is the break your body was looking for to reload its defenses to be stronger for the next battle. And there is always another battle.

It is important that rest (correct meditation does count as rest) and proper nutrition are also included in this paradigm. You must also keep yourself as free from known allergens as possible. We need the recuperation properties of the body to be focused on healing the body with clean oxygen, not fighting off pathogens by releasing huge amount of histamine. Think of armies being divided in too many directions to be effective in defeating an enemy invader. Eventually the defenses will break down and the body will succumb to the allergy/asthma attack.

The next several sections of the book deal with making the body, the physical temple of the mind, a healthy and safe environment. We will focus on nutrition, exercise and, finally, the breathing methods of meditation to give you a game plan to taking back control of your own life.

The Future

As I write this book, scientists are developing an experimental genetically engineered asthma drug that might change the way asthmatics take medications forever! In 1999, the New England Journal of Medicine reported a breakthrough with a new drug, rhuMab-E25. While taking this drug, a quarter of the patients on inhaled corticosteroids were able to stop taking the steroids. One third of the patients who were on oral steroids (probably prednisone) were also able to quit.

RhuMAb-E25 is administered by intravenous injections twice weekly for a period of twelve weeks. The tests resulted in the decline of the antibody IgE, which is responsible for the overproduction of histamine. When an asthmatic or someone with allergic diseases encounters an allergen, histamine can inflame the air passages, which causes further difficulty in breathing. RhuMAb-E25 goes right to the source of the problem and reduces the histamine inflammation. The new drug also has promise for allergic rhinenitis and atopic dermatitis.

The drug is experimental at the time of this writing, with the Food and Drug Administration approval expected in 6 months. The drug is currently produced by splicing a tiny segment of a cloned mouse antibody into a human antibody. Therein could be the problem, in my humble opinion, because when we start mixing such chemical structures between species, playing God if you will, accidents of nature are bound to happen.

Regardless of what utopian drug the drug companies' chemists come out with, there are always side effects. One of the greatest truths is that self-empowerment does not begin with a pill or an inhalator; it begins by taking charge and being responsible for your own day-to-day choices and activities.

1. Healing with Whole Foods; Paul Pitchford; pg 39.
2. Cacioppo & Petty, 1982

CHAPTER 5

Nutrition and Diet

The Truth about Diet

Every morsel of food you chew and every beverage you swallow become the future "tools" for your body to reconstruct, heal and rebalance itself and your emotions. From the serotonin levels in the brain (mood) to performance nutrition in anti-aging, nowhere is nutrition more important than for people with autoimmune disorders, which includes allergies and asthma. I think there is more talk about diets today than in other time in history. Whenever I go to the bookstore, the best-seller list always has one new " How to" book about how to lose weight through diet, or diet and exercise, or how to prevent cancer through diet. Everyone professes to have a "new method" of weight loss and disease control, but the truth is that most are the same old diet plans revisited.

Of the ten leading causes of death in the United States, heart disease, cancer, stroke, and to some extent, diabetes mellitus account for two thirds of the 2 million deaths per year. What is interesting is that all four have a common denominator: diet influences the development of the disease in the top four killers. To say that diet has no influence on our health is ludicrous. For asthmatics and people with allergies, it is even more critical and essential to control.

Food is not only important in the aspect of eating non-allergic food items, but also making sure intake is balanced in its nutrition. Nutrition balance is defined as protein, carbohydrates and fats as well as vitamins, minerals, enzymes, water and antioxidants in correct ratio and quantity to refuel and heal the body. Think of it this way: when you starve yourself all day long and finally get to eat, did you ever notice how fast you eat and the enormous quantity of food you gulp down? Take inventory next time you're eating and in a hurry and you will find that subconsciously you actually overeat! The body (actually the brain) has an innate protection mechanism that cannot be overridden for its survival. This survival mechanism is based on the brain needing blood sugar in order to operate and control all the functions of the body, from hormone regulation to muscle reflexes. The brain will sacrifice the body and even the body's health to secure the brain's own adequate food or blood sugar levels. When you do not eat or do not eat the correct "supplies" for the brain and body to do the work that is demanded of it in its day-to-day activities, there is a hierarchical sacrifice that the body goes through for it means to survive. The brain will start to shut down portions of the body not critical (in its judgment) for survival, *and* the brain will secrete chemical messengers into the body that when you do finally eat, to encourage you to eat until the stomach just absolutely cannot contain any more food. Therefore, we eat fast because we are "starving," eat a huge quantity of food (mostly sugar and carbohydrates), far more than we actually need, and the body stores this extra energy in the form of fat because the body never knows when the next meal in coming. This overindulgence is the way the body protects itself from future "starvation methods or diets" and in some cases inaccurate amounts of proper nutrients. This is why starving yourself by limiting calories to ridiculously low amounts never works long term. The body is smarter than you think in protecting its interests.

We can only manipulate the three macronutrients (protein, fats and carbohydrates) to so many ratios and so many hierarchies. Please keep in mind one universal truth: regardless of what we want to believe or what our friends have success with,

YOU HAVE TO FIND YOUR OWN TRUTH IN DIET.

Selecting between a high protein / low carbohydrate or a low-fat/ high-carbohydrate diet because so and so did and lost 10 pounds or take up any other popular trend in dieting…. is nonsense! This is like the entire world's population trying to squeeze into a couple different shoe sizes without any regard to proper fit!

What works for your friends, your brother, mom or dad will not work optimally for you. You have to experiment, introspect, read, research and explore, and most important give each new diet therapy a fair try. In fact, when you change the way you eat, it takes six weeks for the body to regulate itself and adapt to this new way of eating. Each of us has a unique constitution unlike any other, even our parents, (unless you are an identical twin). Therefore, what one brother can eat and get away with will spell trouble for the other brother.

Incidentally the RDA that is posted on food labels is a mechanism for the federal government to allocate your tax dollars to welfare, WIC and other federally funded programs. It is calculated unilaterally without regard to the elderly, athletes, children and people who are extremely tall or short. It's just a measuring stick to decide what agency gets what monies.

In addition to the static theories of diet from our own culture in the West, I definitely believe that there is an energy that flows from each food we consume. I first thought about this when I would get a feeling about a certain food before I ate it. I would instinctively know if it would flare up an allergic reaction on my skin or not. I really believe that by placing the food to your lips you can almost feel if it feels right for you. Chinese diet therapy as well as Ayurvedic and Tibetan medicinal principals have this kind of theory about food having a resonation or energy to it.

Unlike the average dieter, the asthmatic and the allergic have specific needs that are much more complicated, and require more research, time and energy to find their truth. We have special concerns; we may be allergic to many different groups of foods, such as citrus or wheat, or our digestive system is often compromised. I have found that most digestive aids or vitamins that contain digestive aids such as protease, amylase and lipase do not make a notable difference in digestion. The Chinese herbals, however, do make a tremendous difference and can end gas, bloating, and stomach cramps by strengthening the appropriate Yin organ system (more on this later).

The medication we take can alter the way carbohydrates or fats are handled in the body. For instance, prednisone can alter carbohydrate absorption and Benadryl can cause constipation and difficulty in urination, especially if you have an enlarged prostate. Whew! No wonder most people just give up.

One fact that surprised me is that most physicians that you consult for your asthma/allergy control do not have experience in nutrition. In fact, most physicians do not have more than 6 college credits in nutrition. Ask your physician to send you to a nutritionist, a ND (Naturopathic Doctor), or a qualified registered dietitian who is familiar with allergies. Ask and verify that they have experience of many years before you trust them to recommend foods for you. Experience is always the best teacher in my opinion, regardless of how many diplomas are on the wall, especially when it is your skin (literally) on the line!

Food as part of the solution to healing ourselves is a relatively new concept for Americans. It was not until 1988, that the Surgeon General acknowledged the importance of a good diet and at the same time condemned our style of eating. He also believed that two thirds of all deaths are directly affected by our diet. Powerful statements coming from a man of science!

Above all else, read, talk to people who have been down the same road as you, gain from their experiences. Talk to people on the Internet, most importantly .... *THINK* for yourself. After all, no one knows and lives with your body and your body's reactions like you do. You must be open to all possibilities. Sometimes the very thing we love or grew up eating is the very thing we are allergic to and/or is causing the asthma attacks. Many times we have to find ways to adapt to our allergic limitations.

Many people who come to my clinic with chronic conditions have researched quite thoroughly their particular affliction and are extremely versed in its etiology and the treatment options open to them. I like to call them educated consumers in health care. You have to take a proactive part in your healthcare; be educated so that you can make tough decisions.

Let's review some different diet therapies that you may have not heard of and that have helped me. Keep in mind, your body can and will constantly change its reaction to allergens. Therefore, your diet may need to evolve to keep yourself in balance.

Eat to Live or Live to Eat

Let's begin with some essential basics of eating. First, learn to separate actual hunger from just wanting a certain food item for comfort. Food is a wonderful comfort to all of us. With our high tech transportation systems, we have the luxury of being able to buy just about any food ever produced in any country . The temptation is all around us. The hardest lesson is to learn that food is for fuel and performance; not comfort. Food is a means of survival that enables us to function. Food's nutrients make it a healing modality, like any other therapy we would seek out. Many times the very food we crave is strangely the same food that causes us the grief of allergic reaction.

Feasts and dining go back in history as long as man has lived together in families and communities. We try to replicate the pleasure and comfort of getting together and eating with friends by constantly eating. The act of eating and the support of friends become Pavlovian through time and conditioning. At work when we are frustrated, we eat a cookie or go the vending machine and consume something chemically processed. At night when we are disappointed about something or someone, we reach for a slice of cake and milk or munch on the candy that we had in the cabinet.

There is nothing wrong with occasionally reaching for a treat to soothe ourselves. However, when it becomes a compulsion or a vehicle to escape from dealing with life's problems on a daily basis, then you may have to get professional help. Many people get stuck in a pattern of eating the same Oreos and milk every night because of their frustration or disappointment. For those of us who are allergic to so many foods, this can be a deadly combination for allergic reactions or to your overall health.

Most times when we break down and have that little treat; it is the first couple of bites we only really taste and marvel at the taste and texture. After that, the hand and mouth action go on autopilot and the joy of actually tasting the food gives way to the action of just eating. Soon the act of eating, rather than the food itself, becomes the comfort we desire. Therefore when in a miserable state, we want to prolong that feeling of comfort, so we eat longer, consume larger and larger portions, and our waistline begins to expand.

Try to think of food as one of your therapies, just like your medicine. When you are packing your lunch and snacks for work, make healthy choices according to your nutritional needs as well as your allergen needs. Reserve special times for eating "the guilt foods" when you are with family or friends or on a special occasion. Make the whole experience unique and positive, from the food to the company.

According to Chinese Medicine food therapy, it is believed that greasy and/or sweet food may injure the Spleen (one of the 5 Yin organs -more about this in Chapter 12) by creating mucous and heat in the body. Sugar, milk and cheese should also be avoided. Many children have an allergic reaction to cow's milk. I lived on goat's milk for twenty years. We all know that we consume far too much sugar in America, so reducing the amount of sugar and saturated fat we consume can only help us in a multitude of ways.

For those of you who are on corticosteroids (prednisone) to control their asthma or allergies carbohydrates are a special concern. Your body is not able to break down carbohydrates as well as other people. You will have a tendency to store more fat and water than normal. For people like us, the ratio of fat, carbohydrate and protein is of utmost importance. This ratio may have to fluctuate a bit because of your allergies. For instance, if you are a person who is allergic to fish, chicken, and nuts (quite common), your variety of protein becomes instantly hampered.

Macronutrient Ratio

For people like us, the importance of protein cannot be emphasized enough. Your ratio of protein, from various sources, should be around 40% of calories. Your carbohydrates should weigh in around 45%, and 15% should be left for fat. Your saturated fat should be as low as you can tolerate; around 5% is good. Your saturated fats should come from a good source, such as salmon or mackerel if you are not allergic to it.

Meals should be eaten frequently and often; ideally as many as eight to ten times a day with a minimum of four. Try to space extremely small meals out at intervals every two or three hours, as this is easier on your body. Not just from the perspective of digestion and keeping the blood sugar levels more stable and consistent; but it is easier on the immune system to handle small quantities of allergens than huge amounts - especially if you eat something mistakenly that you are allergic to.

Eggs, for example, are a common allergen, and are used as an ingredient in everything from baked goods to sauces. Many foods can sneak up on you like this. Every time you have dinner with friends or acquaintances, eat at business meetings or try a new restaurant or ethnic food, you are at risk.

One final tip. Try to eat foods uncommon to your ethnic background. If you are Eastern European, try eating Chinese, Japanese or Indian food. I found that this has worked for me. I lived on turkey and rice for years when I was a child, as it was uncommon for my ancestors to eat this kind of food and therefore develop an allergy to it. As we know, allergic reactions can change and will change in time. Make sure that you experiment with food when you can control the variables of preparation and selection.

Protein

Beans of all types and preparations, legumes and seeds, and nuts, if you can tolerate them round out your protein choices. Meat is always the first thing to come to mind when we say protein. Deer meat (venison) is also an excellent low fat choice for people with allergies. Turkey is usually well tolerated, as well as duck (although it is greasy if not prepared correctly). Some of the tofu that has herbal flavorings isn't bad either. If you have Multiple Chemical Sensitivity (MCS), try to get organic meat.

I have found that an animal's frequency of fertility has a lot to do with allergic reactions. For instance, chickens are constantly fertile (ability to lay eggs) whereas ducks are fertile only seasonally. A person allergic to chicken or chicken eggs will probably not be allergic to duck or duck eggs. It has to do with the hormones flowing through the fowl's bloodstream.

Carbohydrates

Carbohydrates, or carbs, are a problem for many people these days. I don't think that carbohydrates make you fat, nor does any other macronutrient. The problem is the preponderance of carbohydrates that are out there today. Potato chips, corn chips, pizzas, and the fructose sweetener in so many of our drinks (including adding additional high fructose syrup to fruit drinks) are the main culprits. We are bombarded with snacks and staples that are predominantly carbohydrate. It is only natural that majorities of our calories come from carbohydrate and fat additives.

Whenever I wonder whether I should eat something that is "hot" or trendy, I go back to basics. In a world of supplemental wizardry, it is very easy these days to make something so scientific and complicated and sell it to the public in a fancy container with the words 'scientific breakthrough" plastered on it. It is incredibly difficult to sell something on simplicity alone, as it has to stand on its own merits. Given today's engineered foods and supplements, aggressive marketing, and our quest for something better, we constantly try new foods with additives to give us nutritional value. For example, think of all the "meal replacement" bars and shakes and the plethora of info-mercials selling late night products.

For the allergically challenged, of which I qualify, simple is always better. The closer to the way nature produced and packaged the nutrient, the better. Moreover, in that same line of thinking, the simpler the food the better the body will be able to digest it and break it down properly. Try not to make your diet any more complicated than it is already with your food limitations.

Basically, carbohydrates can be broken down into two groups: simple and complex. Try to provide your body with grains (complex carbohydrates) with the husk and fiber intact (whole grains). Eat two to three servings of whole grains per day. Whole grains will keep you living longer by fighting heart disease, blocking cancer, keeping diabetes at bay and (here is the bonus:) allowing you to lose weight. The simple carbohydrates come from fruits with the skin intact, which contain necessary fiber and pectin, and natural sugars such as honey.

Whole grains are defined as having four components: The husk or chaff, the bran or outer layer, the endosperm or the bulk of the grain, and the germ or the core. A whole grain food contains at least 51% whole grain by weight. Modern processing removes the bran and/or the germ and retails it back to you as a separate product. Two of my favorite whole grains are buckwheat and kasha. There is also wild and brown rice, bulgur wheat, oats (oatmeal old fashioned), cracked wheat, amaranth, popcorn, triticale, barley, flax, buckwheat, rye, couscous, and quinoa (pronounced "keenwa").

Contrary to popular belief, white rice, cornmeal and whole kernel corn are not whole grains. Many people, when speaking of grains, think immediately of cereal. Some of the better choices with more than 90% whole grains are: shredded wheat, slow cooked oatmeal, Cheerios, and Wheaties. Check the manufacturers label for "whole grain" on the box and see it has the word "whole" in its ingredients list, such as "whole oats" or "whole rye." In addition try to get product marked GMO free or non genetically modified, as I believe that this will be a future problem with allergically sensitive people.

Understand that as a person with allergies/asthma, many of these "whole" products may create more of a reaction than their watered down cousins when one is allergic to them.

Journaling

One of the most helpful tools for you, which can also help your doctor, is journaling. Journaling is simply writing things down about your day and your experiences that give a timeline that helps you or your health care provider to figure out what is triggering asthma attacks or allergic reactions. Most of us cannot remember in detail what we ate 48 hours ago, but it is that very food/trigger that you forgot about that can make your body go into a histamine hissy fit. Many times we do not track our emotional outbursts, worry or anger for example, that we keep pent up inside of us leading to overeating or worse.

Please keep in mind that the body works in cycles of action to reaction to action. Inside, our bodies are in constant movement, adjustment, action and reaction. They are never still and quiet even when in the deepest of sleep. Movement is life. Movement or action is both internal and external, Yin and Yang.

This movement can range from a chemical reaction via a chemical messenger relay system that says that a particle is a foreign invader and I will sneeze to get it out of my body, to the panicky thoughts one can have about an exam which upset our stomach to the point that we can't eat. Movement is also the jog that you took this morning and all the adjustments to heart rate and respiration that were made along the way, as well as to the extra filtration of air that had to go during that jog as your body tried to purify the air the best way it could do.

All that we eat, emotionally feel, physically move and think about affects us in some way and definitely affects the delicate balance of the body's internal adjustment systems. Later when we explain what Yin and Yang theory is in Chinese Medicine, you will see how the ancients might have had a better grasp on the true mechanics of the body than we currently do with our segregated systems of diagnoses.

The body is cyclic in nature, and just one thing can make the delicate system start to wobble out of its normal circular pattern.

Air Passages: Nutrition and Diet

Day:	SATURDAY		
TIME	**ACTIVITY**	**EMOTIONS**	**PHYSICAL**
7am	Woke. Ate: 2 eggs fired in a little olive oil; 1 slice wheat toast; coffee with skim milk		Head stuffy. Full of mucous. Slight headache
8am	Hand washed car. New car soap		Hands red and itchy
9am	Walk with neighbor. Strong perfume smell		
11 am	Showered with Ivory Soap		
11:30 – 1:30	Went to office; filing in dusty area	Stayed longer than I wanted – ANGRY	Wheezy; used Albuterol
1:30 – 2:30	Home & Lunch; 2 cups coffee; non dairy creamer; grilled chicken salad w/ oil & vinegar dressing		
3:30 – 4:00	Nap	Dreamed in vivid color of being chased	Refreshed
4:00 – 6:30	Cleaned house: Windex; Endust; Mop-n-Glow		No problems
6:30	Showered – Ivory soap; Head & Shoulders shampoo		Tired
8:00 – 10:00 pm	Dinner: 1 glass merlot; lobster bisque soup; sourdough bread; stuffed sole with crabmeat; chocolate mousse	Happy and relaxed	Stuffy; used nasal spray
10:00 pm	Dancing!		
1:30 am	Bed		Stuffy and slight headache

In the truest sense of the word, all that health care professionals do to heal is to try to figure out what went wrong in the balance of the body and what is the quickest way to return it to a normal state of balance. The best way to help figure out this mystery is to keep track of all the minute details of your day .

Parents, if you are journaling for your child, this will be a lot harder, especially if they are in daycare, school, or go over to a friend's house. If you really want to play detective, try to get the cooperation of the school teacher; ask what activities they did that day. Perhaps they used a different brand of glue or paste; ask to see the ingredients list. Many times something simple like glue or paint can cause chemical problems for a child with allergic sensitivity, especially if the child is exposed over long parts of the day or succeeding days.

Before we go on to detoxifying the body, please start to journal a week or two before the actual detox plan goes into effect. This will establish a baseline on how your body is coping before, during, and after the detox. This is valuable information for someone like me who sits down with his clients and their completed journals for several hours and figures out what is going on.

Chinese Diet Therapy

The whole concept of Chinese Medicine is intriguing to me. The science of Chinese Medicine has only recently been tested, not only here in the U.S., but around the world. The National Institutes of Health is spending more time in analyzing the Chinese health system, and finding that it is a very practical, cost efficient way of managing the health of one of the largest populations on Earth.

I will try to explain Chinese Diet therapy without too much Chinese terminology and to put it into laymen's terms, but understand that it is a science unto its own. The Chinese divide foods by their properties of Five Flavors and Five Temperatures that correspond to the Five Elements (see Chapter 11 for further detail).

Air Passages: Nutrition and Diet

The Five Flavors are:

> Salty for the Kidneys
> Sour for the Liver
> Bitter for the Heart
> Sweet for the Spleen
> Pungent for the Lungs

Thus asthmatics should consume pungent foods for the Lungs. Pungent foods include garlic, onions, ginger, chilies and cinnamon. These foods perform several functions, including:

> Clearing the Lungs of mucous
> Improving digestion (associated with Spleen injury common in asthma/allergies)
> Stimulating blood circulation and cardiovascular health
> Improving Liver function
> Warming, relaxing and moistening the Kidneys, thus preventing adrenal burnout

It is interesting in Chinese Medicine, each of the five Yin organs represent the five flavors (Liver, Heart, Kidneys, Spleen and Lungs) can be controlled by the energy, called postnatal Qi, that we consume (food, water and air).

The Five Temperatures of food are Hot, Warm, Neutral, Cool and Cold. This has nothing to do with the temperature that the food is served at, but rather its inherent property. Each of these divisions then has a Yin or Yang property assigned to them as well.

Unlike the West, diets are not divided into "Good foods" or "Bad foods," or protein, carbohydrates and fats. Diets are assigned based on your genetic constitution and your environment, which is further broken down into external environment and internal environment. Here's an example of how external environmental changes affect health and healing: if you are from Minnesota and you take a vacation to the Caribbean in January, your body, in order to compensate, may drive you to crave and consume too many cold or cooling foods, which is Yin. The end result is that you may end up with diarrhea. (no pun intended!)

External environment can also be the season of year; you should adjust the foods consumed to that particular time of the year. For example, in the Autumn, you should reinforce and moisten Lung

Qi by consuming more fruits and by preparing for Winter by strengthening the Kidneys with consumption of root vegetables and seeds.

An example of imbalance in the internal environment would be the symptoms of an allergic reaction: inflammation and heat, excessive thirst and low tolerance for high humidity. A Chinese Doctor might prescribe foods that are more cooling, such as bean sprouts and eggplant and suggest eliminating food such as onions, and would thus be pungent (Lung element) that will be drying and create more heat.

HOT	WARM	NEUTRAL	COOL	COLD
Black Pepper	Leeks	Shitaki Mushrooms	Eggplant	Watermelon
Green Pepper	Coconuts	Peanuts	Bean Sprouts	Water Chestnuts
Cinnamon	Sunflower Seeds	Figs	Soy	Tomatoes

Attention to food and its direct effect on the internal organs is a very intrinsic part of the therapies provided by the physicians in China. It would serve us well to heed their recommendations.

Obviously, these concepts could fill a whole book, but being aware of them may help you to understand valuable options when you look outside the box in treating your own allergies/asthma. One of the services I have found extremely useful for my clients is customized Chinese eating plans for their allergies and asthma.

Sugar is a Food for Cancer

Although I have never met anyone allergic to sugar cane or table sugar, I am sure it is possible. Americans are consuming over 43 teaspoons of pure sugar a day (an average of 130 pounds per person per year) with 40% of their diet coming from the wrong kinds of fats (hydrogenated, saturated and fractured). A 1995 study showed that sugar taken on an empty stomach could lead to an inability to concentrate. This type of diet creates disease in the body.

One of the most astounding cancer related discoveries occurred in the late nineteen seventies. Emanuel Cheraskin, MD demonstrated that a single ingestion of sugar could lower the phagocytic activity (destruction and consumption of foreign invaders) of white blood cells for up to five hours. With immune defenses lowered, cancer cells, which are in the body constantly, can run amok. In other correlated studies, glucotoxicity (high blood glucose) has been shown to double the risk of rectum, colon, breast, ovary, prostrate and pancreatic cancer. In fact, PET (positive emission tomography) scans in hospitals all over the world detect cancer cells by imaging the feeding frenzy that goes on as cancer consumes the deposits of glucose.

Cancer cells primarily use glucose via the anaerobic glycolytic pathway. Hepatomas and fibrosarcomas cells using as much as .60 gm of glucose for growth. Carcinomas consuming twice that amount [1] In addition, glucotoxicity may lower immune functions by preventing neutrophils (white blood cells that are attracted to inflammation) to phagocyze (eat) bacteria. Starch did not have this effect at all [2].

With that in mind, the most effective Healing Cancer Diet uses an alkaline food base of low glycemic index (GI) foods in their raw state or only slightly cooked or steamed (Qi intact). I have developed and used this type of diet extensively in my clinic to help stabilize cancer clients as well as to assist people with diabetes mellitus, obesity, and severe allergies and asthma.

Low Glycemic Index Foods

Eating low glycemic index foods is important because allergies and asthma cause a huge amount of stress on the body. Stress can be defined as when demand(s) exceeds the body's coping abilities (i.e., allergens or fear of lack of air driving the asthma attack) Stress causes everything from hypersensitivity reaction (an asthma attack) to eczema, neurodermititis, and even acne. When under stress, the body is not able to handle well the foods that need to be immediately broken down, because the liver floods the body with blood sugar and the stomach increases gastric secretions. Low GI foods that trickle through the digestive system will not throw the body into an emergency state caused by having to handle large surges in blood sugar.

The glycemic index is not new. It was developed in 1981 by Dr. David Jenkins, a professor of nutrition at the University of Toronto, who wanted to devise a carbohydrate safe diet for people with diabetes. Interestingly enough, the very insulin imbalances that were causing diabetes also were being linked to an insulin/cancer relationship. It has been well documented that insulin, a major anabolic hormone in mammals, is involved in malignancies [3].

The glycemic index measures pure glucose, which elevates blood sugar levels to an assigned 100 points. All foods are then assigned a value in relation to their effect on blood sugar levels (glucose) coming as close to 100 as possible. For example, cherries have a GI of 22, whereas watermelon has a GI of 72. High GI foods have a rating of above 70. Low GI foods have values below 55. Choose foods below 65, if possible, when you select carbohydrates.

But it's more complicated than just finding a food's GI number. There are so many varieties of foods from mushrooms to rice. Rice for example, is a major staple of many Asian countries and its popularity is rising in America as well. Rice varies in its glycemic index by the amount of amylose (a starch) that it contains. The higher the amylose, the lower the glycemic index. A typical guideline is if the rice is "sticky," then it has low amylose and therefore a higher GI rating.

Examples of foods with low GI include: roasted peanuts (15), Uncle Ben's Converted rice (44), old fashioned oatmeal (49), apples (38), whole grain pumpernickel bread (51), and navy bean soup (38).

Asthma and pH

PH is a term thrown out there a lot in the last year, but it is nothing new to Naturopaths and the way they treat all disease. PH is a medium to measure, on a graduated scale, the hydrogen in the body (pH = potential hydrogen). The lower the pH number the greater the amount of acidity in the body, and the higher the pH, the greater the alkalinity.

"Jin Ye" is the term used in Chinese Medicine for the two kinds of fluids in the body. Jin is the fluids that define blood, but can include all mucous membranes, sweat and urine and the fluid in your eyes. The Jin in the eyes is important because the cornea has no blood supply and is nourished with life- giving oxygen by that very fluid that keeps it moist. The Ye is all the other fluids such as lymphatic fluid, cerebrospinal fluid, and the humor lubricating the joints

To be clear, I have used the two concepts of Jin Ye and pH exclusively in my practice for the last 5 years to regulate everything from cancer to fibromyalgia to allergies. Most Americans eating a diet of pasta, chocolate, beef, coffee and tea, beer and wine, eggs and bread, can produce acidic fluid levels in the body that can lead to disruption of normal body processes. PH is so important for regulation in the blood that sliding up and down the pH scale just 1 point can lead to instant death! Just as acid rain destroys a pristine forest or excess alkalinity can pollute a lake and kill fish, imbalance of pH slowly compromises cellular integrity in our own bodies.

PH is so important that the body has developed strict accounting procedures to monitor acid/alkaline balances in every cell of your body (comprised mostly of fluid) and in the 60,000 miles of the blood's transportation mechanisms. Remember that the blood carries life-supporting oxygen that touches everything in your body that needs healing or repairing and also removes carbon dioxide that can become toxic. If the body has a hard time maintaining homeostasis in the blood (proper pH around 7.34 to 7.4), the whole body feels like it is under attack. Extreme variances in pH can kill us. Extremely acidic individuals will hold onto fat (obesity) as a method to diffuse the toxic acid across a larger surface area, thus aiding in the survival of the organism.

Fundamentally, all regulation systems - including breathing, digestion, hormonal production, and circulation - all depend on the bodys ability to regulate pH by removing metabolized acid residues without damaging the cells in the body tissue.

Proper pH balance will:

> Correct fat metabolism and weight control along with healthy insulin production.
>
> Allow smooth blood flow and regulation of blood pressure.
>
> Stimulate cellular regeneration and DNA/RNA synthesis necessary for recovery from disease.
>
> Regulate calcium utilization to lessen osteoporosis and osteoarthritis.

There are only two ways that we can actively control pH levels in our body: our eating patterns and our breathing patterns. If our choices in food are incorrect, then the kidneys will have to filter out the excess phosphates and sulfates to stabilize the body to normal pH levels. Over time this can place an enormous strain on the kidneys. Remember this when we begin our discussion of Chinese Medical QiGong. If we become too acidic we will pass out. Hence the body's way of compensating is hyperventilation or breathing too rapidly or with shallow breaths very quickly.

The chemical equation that explains all respiration and acid/base balance is as follows:

$$H_2O + CO_2 \Longleftrightarrow H_2CO_3 \Longleftrightarrow H^+ \Longrightarrow HCO_3$$

You can monitor your body's pH level with pH strips. They are an easy and convenient way to measure pH level. The morning pH after sleeping all night, should be slightly lower (6.5) as this is after not eating at all for 6-8 hours. The pH after meals should be around 7.2 - 7.4, if you are eating the correct balance of foods.

Eating Patterns and pH Regulation

Before you select what to eat you must have an idea of what your average pH is over several days, as it does fluctuate. We use two types of tests in our office: a saliva test and urine strip test to measure what pH your body carries. Once we know what your potential is, we construct a custom dietary program for you to follow (allergic interaction's are considered). I also use Chinese dietary therapy as an adjunct to pH to further balancing out the Yin and Yang properties of foods as well. Good examples of raw alkaline forming foods are carrots, beets, miso soup, raw goats milk, buckwheat and sour cherries. In addition, one should consume as much of the following foods as possible for detoxification: Rhubarb and its stems, blueberries, Swiss chard, radishes, kohlrabi, apples, and grapes. Incidentally, apples and grapes have a low glycemic index when eaten raw and with skins.

What this shift in food selection accomplishes in chemical terms is a transition from an acid-based diet to an alkaline-based diet. Cancer cells thrive in an acid-based environment, with the proliferation of cancer cells inversely proportional to an alkaline state of the blood. The pH level of the blood is actually a measurement of hydrogen. When the pH is high, which means there are too many hydrogen atoms, then the blood will become more acidic. High acid based diets produce more phosphorus, sulfur, chlorine and iodine while alkaline-based diets produce more calcium, magnesium, potassium and sodium.

Acid forming foods, with their tendency to promote mucous and acidosis, create a more hostile environment in the body. This is especially true in the tender state of cancer or severe allergies. Some raw foods that are acid-forming that should be avoided include sauerkraut, eggs, alcohol, pasteurized milk, prunes and some medical drugs. The best way to measure the body's acid/alkaline balance is measurement of the urine and saliva over a 24 hour period.

Breathing Patterns and pH Regulation

Since breathing is an important factor in pH regulation, and actually affects pH more than the food you eat, this obviously is an important consideration. Stress in our daily lives contributes enormously to pH deregulation and a host of other catalytic problems. Medical QiGong uses slow and disease-specific exercise prescriptions along with individualized breathing techniques to reach the desired goal of pH regulation. Medical QiGong exercises have been used for over 5 thousand years for this purpose and have endured the test of time and efficacy. I have found that Medical QiGong is critically important in the regulation of Asthma, cancer, CFS (chronic fatigue syndrome), fibromyalgia, panic disorders and even panic disorder linked with obsessive-compulsive disorder. (More about QiGong in Chapter 13.)

In a severe asthma attack, the pH often begins to drop, which can lead to respiratory acidosis and even death. One old remedy I have used uses common household items to alleviate an asthma attack is baking soda in a glass of regular ginger ale. This does two things:

> 1. The ginger ale, when drunk quickly has a tendency to make you belch; this always seemed to help in my asthma attack. In fact I could always tell when my asthma attack was subsiding or easing up because I usually belched.
>
> 2. The baking soda dissolved in the ginger ale brings the pH balance back to alkaline, reversing the severity of acidosis.

Since I have also used plain baking soda under the tongue sublingually this diffuses into the capillary beds quite quickly and does not have to pass through the digestive tract. Do not use this method all the time, though.

As our diet in the western world continually goes through revision of faster food preparation and less enzyme-producing food coming from raw sources, and as our stress levels increase and promote irregular breathing patterns that we might not be aware of, attention to pH regulation should be part of everyone's daily health routine.

The Raw Food Diet for Asthma / Allergy patients

Raw foods are foods that are bioelectrically still active, or in Chinese terms that have robust and healthy Qi within them. Said another way, the electrical charge between cells and within cells is still active and vibrant. This cellular activity has the ability to remove toxins at a higher rate and maintain the bodies capacity to regulate nutrients and oxygen within the cells themselves. Research from the First Medical Clinic at the University of Vienna has found that a live food diet increases the microelectrical potential of tissues and can restore previous cellular degeneration that has lost its electrical potential. Said another way, raw food can heal tissue.

Kirlian photography is a useful tool to measure the bioelectric fields of live foods as well as human beings. The stronger the life force of a cell, the stronger and brighter the electroluminescence of a Kirlian photographic field, which corresponds to the electrical potential of the sum of cells photographed.

By measuring foods before and after cooking or processing, we can visibly see how the Qi is affected, how much life force we are placing in our bodies, and, in turn, how much healing potential that food has.

Preparation of Food

When we compare Chinese and Western diets, we find several unique distinctions. For example, the people of China consume more than 20% *more* calories per day than we do in the United States, yet there seems to be little obesity or malnutrition (4).

The Chinese consume three times as much fiber as Americans do and consume less than half of the fat. Their blood cholesterol values are half of their American counterparts and they suffer from far less colon and rectal cancer.

Interesting differences between Chinese and American diets include the fact that in China vegetables and meats are cooked together, and the portion size of meat and fish is considered small by American standards. The drinking of tea (green or black) or soup is included in the meal. The Chinese include a tremendous variety of vegetables in each meal rather than one or maybe two vegetables in the American dinner or supper. Cooking in a wok uses far less oil (a tablespoon or two) for the entire family than the copious use of hydrogenated cooking oils in U.S. fast food restaurants. In addition, the gelatinization or swelling of starch (rice) is not as great in wok cooking, and therefore the glycemic index will not increase as it does with other methods of cooking.

The Chinese cut all foods into small bite size pieces, which require less cooking time and destroy less vital nutrients (Qi). The cooking water is not thrown away but is allowed to soak up into the rice that later is consumed with all the vital life force intact.

Keeping the life force potential in food also means being careful about food preparation methods. Here is a ranking of food preparation methods according to their ability to retain the vital life force (Qi) of food:

- Raw
- Wok cooking
- Steaming
- Pressure cooking or boiling
- Deep-frying
- Barbecue and grilling
- Oven baking
- Microwave cooking

Food Additives

With so much processing of foods today for the sake of time and convenience, sometimes we really do not know what we are eating. Couple that with the vast amount of food imported from other countries; that do not always adhere to our food safety protocols, and this can spell trouble for someone with asthma or allergies.

President Clinton established the President's Council of Food Safety in 1999 to act as a watchdog and prohibit the import of unsafe food into the United States. Many times in the past, importers rejected in one port and would "shop" around until they could be accepted in another. Now the cargo will clearly be marked as "Refused US." This ought to make those of us who are sensitive and allergic to chemicals sleep a little better.

A couple of terms that you may see associated with food additive allergies are:

Urticaria: also called hives, this is a temporary condition identified by itching and edema in patches.

Angioedema: A swelling, puffy, flushing response caused by fluids rushing into the tissues.

Anaphylaxis: a general allergic reaction marked by difficulty in breathing, wheezing and a shock-like state. Many times this is reported to happen in the throat.

There is a list produced by the FDA called the GRAS (Generally Recognized As Safe) list, which contains all food additives that are generally recognized as safe. The list dates back to 1958. A good place to check for information is the federal web site vm.cfsan.fda.gov/~lrd/foodadd.html. This could be a full time job for several people because the FDA certified over 11.5 million pounds of color additives in 1995 alone!

The FDA divides food coloring into two groups. One is certified by the batch of petroleum and coal sources it comes from. The other is exempt from batch certification which comes from plant, animal or mineral sources such as fruit juices, carmine and titanium dioxide.

Although the FDA is concerned about food to additives and their effects on people's health, it takes quite a few complaints before starting any investigation, removing the substance from the GRAS list, or funding research on the product. Allergies and asthma are such fickle things that sometimes it is very difficult to know what is to blame for your misery. By the time an allergen is isolated, a lot of effort, time and even money has been spent, and that is just for one sensitivity.

My advice is what the doctors told me long ago when I was a child, "be your own best detective".

MSG

Probably the biggest demon for me and many others is the MSG additive that is so famous in oriental cooking. In fact, it was so notorious for causing discomfort that the reaction it causes became known as Chinese restaurant syndrome. Allergic symptoms I have heard of include headaches, facial flushing, weakness, heart palpitations, irritability, depression and, of course, a topical rash. Usually the symptoms start within 10 to 15 minutes of consumption and can last for hours, or days in the case of itching or rash.

Monosodium glutamate, or MSG, also goes by the alias "hydrolyzed vegetable protein" or HVP and sometimes just as "flavoring" in many ingredient lists.

Cochineal

This is a red colorant is harvested by extracting the pigment off female cochineal bugs in Central and South America. The bugs are propagated specifically producing the dye contained in food, drinks, cosmetics and fibers of different shades of red, orange, pink and purple.

This substance is listed as "cochineal extract" or "carmine dye" on most labels, but can also be listed as "color added", "artificial color" or "artificial color added".

Cochineal has long been suspected of causing anaphylactic shock, but never confirmed because the standard testing used by many allergists (RAST) does not support the extract.

If we take a look at anything that our kids are eating (and ourselves perhaps) from the candy to the newest beverage sensation, the more electrifying the color the better it sells. They have even changed the color of ketchup now!

Yellow #5

Yellow #5 is widely used in foods, prescription drugs, cosmetics, and even surgical sutures and contact lenses. It can cause itching or hives, but anyone who has extensive allergy sensitivities should be cautious.

It is listed as "tartrazine" in medicine labels, or FD&C Yellow No. 5. The FDA certifies about two millions pounds of this color annually!

Red #3

This is probably one of the most controversial color additives in existence. The FDA applied the Delaney clause in 1990 to outlaw the use of strawberry-toned FD&C #3 in cosmetics and externally applied drugs. Also known as erythrosine, Red 3 in large amounts has been shown in studies to cause thyroid tumors in rats.

The dye is found in bubble gum, maraschino cherries, baked goods, and all kinds of candy and drugs. Like its cousin red #2, red #3 may eventually be banned due to public outcry.

1.) Gullino,PM,Cancer Research,vol27,p1031,June1967
2.) Sanchez, A, Amer.J.Clin.Nutr., vol26,pg1180,Nov1983
3.) Yam, D., Medical Hypothesis, vol.38,p.111,1992
4.) L. Roberts, Diet and health in China, Science 240 (1988)

CHAPTER 6

Detoxification and Supplementation

Creating a Detoxification Plan

Once you are so overwhelmed with allergic reaction that no therapy seems to be of value, it is time to cut your losses and start fresh. By this I mean that the body is in such a state of circular disrepair - awash with histamines and chemical reactions that ignite another chemical reaction etc. - that everything that you do or try seems to aggravate the symptoms further. This is the time to start fresh and clean out the system with a detox method that will allow the body to stabilize and calm itself down.

The bombardment of allergic foods, pharmaceuticals that we ingest, pollution that we breathe, coupled with the lack of nutritive support in the correct ratios, impaired digestion, and compromised immune function all gang up on the body till it begins to shut down and become allergic to everything. At this point it is hard to deduce what is truly causing the allergic reaction. When you are in this state, it is imperative that you address it properly.

The most successful way that I have accomplished this with my clients as well as myself is through a very simple diet plan that includes only a couple of foods, plenty of water, rest and meditation. I first learned of detoxification when I was young and hospitalized for several weeks during which I was only allowed black tea with a little bit of sugar and complete bed rest. Needless to say, I dropped an incredible amount of weight (now I know that I lost huge amounts of muscle and bone density as well) and was weak as a kitten, but my skin did clear for the first time in months.

Understand that in order to detox completely, you need to rest and reduce your stress load to at least half of what you consider normal for you. You need to do this in order to avoid inciting the "flight or fight" response when you are trying to rid your body of chemical toxins. If you can, take a week off work and nurture yourself. If you think about it, for many of us the commute alone really stresses us out even before our day begins. This is a heck of a way to start an eight to ten hour workday!

Air Passages: Detoxification and Supplementation

Hopefully, you have good support mechanisms in place around you, including your spouse, roommate or parents etc. who will comfort and encourage you during this critical time. If you are not in a supportive environment, try to go somewhere that is. This is to be a new beginning for you and you must try to make it as comfortable and painless as possible.

Once you have a nurturing and supportive environment, you can begin to let your body heal. Next, select your menu of simple foods to prepare for your detox plan. For the first couple of days, stick to a liquid fast that will allow the digestive system to rest and will quickly encourage the inflammation to subside.

A few basics first, before going on a juice fast or a detox plan. Ease into it by changing your diet for a few weeks. Namely, avoid all saturated (solid at room temperature), polyunsaturated and hydrogenated fats; refined flour and sugar; all alcohol and caffeine, all processed and prepackaged foods with their preservatives; and excessive animal protein (no more than 4 oz. per day). Absolute no-nos are processed colas and soft drinks, especially anything with aspartame in it. This will prepare your body for cleansing.

Additionally, in order to facilitate a complete cleaning of the intestinal tract and to kill any parasites that may exist in the tract itself, consume 3 oz. of raw rice every morning before eating anything else. Just place it in your mouth and chew and chew and chew, until it is masticated so well and you have generated enough saliva from chewing that you can swallow it. In addition take a good liver supplement that contains the following: turmeric, dandelion extract, milk thistle (80% silymarin). Include an activated charcoal supplement of 500 mg. three times per day 1-2 hours before meal and medication. This will bind intestinal toxins and excrete them in the stool.

After this initial preparation of a few weeks, we are now ready to move on to the juice fast. The recipe for the juice fast is simple. Depending on your sensitivity, select a beverage such as cranberry juice or apple juice, (abstain from citrus at this point). Mix the juice with equal parts noncarbonated water in a 12 oz. glass. If you are not allergic to the following, this is my favorite tasting alkaline juice concoction: pineapple juice (the bromalein in pineapple is an antiinflammatory), apple, Concorde grape, apricot, and papaya. Papaya actually cleans mucous out of the intestinal tract. You may also add a scoop of protein powder. You will sip this throughout the day (at least every half hour) to sustain glucose (blood sugar) levels to the brain and include as many glasses of water as you can tolerate. This diluted fructose (simple sugar from fruit) is very easy on the digestive system and is typically very benign in so far as allergic sensitivity. Again, stay on this juice plan for one to two days and severely limit physical activity and get plenty of rest.

Optionally, you can alternate the juice in your fast with the following alkaline vegetable broth that is high in minerals, unless of course you have allergies to the ingredients:

        2 cups carrots tops
        2 cups beet tops
        2 cups red skinned potato peeling 1/2 inch thick
        3 cups celery stock w/ tops
        several sprigs of parsley
        2 quarts distilled water

Chop all the ingredients very finely and place them in a stainless steel pot with the water. Bring the broth to a boil, place a lid on the pot and simmer on low heat for 20 minutes. Strain and sip. This will keep in the refrigerator for the length of your 2 day fast.

Rest from my perspective, is NOT "just" throwing a load of laundry in or "just" cutting the front part of the lawn, Rest is NOT washing the floor nor running the sweeper, and is not riding your bike or climbing trees. It means to read something pleasurable, meditate, sleep or watch a favorite movie. Allow your mind to heal as well as your body. Better yet, when is the last time that you had total silence in your environment for more than an hour? Silence can be very nurturing to the psyche and the body and most of us have forgotten what that term actually means.

After juice fasting for a maximum of two days, move on to the next step of the detox plan: consuming solid food again. The menu is simple. Pick two foods that are as allergically benign as possible for you. Two combinations that I recommend are a meal of organic turkey and beets or organic lamb and wild rice. The portions should be very small at each sitting, only 1 to 2 oz. of turkey or lamb at a time with a tablespoon of beets or wild rice. The key here is to consume very small meals and to have these meals six times per day. I know that this sounds like a punishment, but your body will thank you for this when you are done. Stay on this for a minimum of 5 more days.

While you are on the 5-day solid food portion of this diet, I highly recommend that you practice QiGong, taichiquan or some form of gentle stretching to invigorate the blood and the lymphatic system. The body is not designed to be motionless for long periods of time and you will stiffen and tighten and feel much worse instead of better if you do not move the blood around a little. A good plan is to do QiGong (more on this later) or stretch upon rising in the morning, then eat your meal and follow it by taking a nap or reading.

We often hear of juice fasts and their wonderful rejuvenating properties. I have found that for most of us with allergies and asthma, the detox timetable is quite lengthy, but to stay on a juice fast longer than a week is ludicrous for our active life-styles today. I find my two-day juice detox and 5-days of benign food works best.

Once you have eliminated all the toxins from your body, given it plenty of rest and begin to add one food at a time to your meal plan. Continue with this food for a week or so, and take note of your reactions (see Chapter 5 on Journaling). Additionally, at the end of the week of new food introduction, you may include a juice fast for 2 days, followed by foods that you are allergically stable with for 5 days etc.

Liver Stabilization Through Diet

I have found that by the time most people look to natural methods of healing, they have already tried many other avenues of allopathic treatment, specifically pharmaceutical drugs. In allergic disorders, there obviously has been a consistent, and sometimes-violent, reaction to something the body treats as a poison, even though that trigger may be a common food. All these past 'poisons' have a good chance of building up and creating a domino effect of symptoms ranging from bloating and weight gain, to mood changes and headaches, to chronic fatigue, high blood pressure and hypoglycemia. In order to start the body on its healing journey, often we have to look at the liver function and stabilize the body's chemistry.

One of the ways to stabilize the body's chemistry is stabilization of the liver itself. The liver, looked at from the Chinese Medicine

Air Passages: Detoxification and Supplementation

viewpoint or the western medical viewpoint, is paramount for the continued detoxification of the blood and body. Without the functions of liver, one would die within several days. Keeping the liver healthy and functional is vital to the recuperation of all immune suppressed patients.

One of the most important functions of the liver is the secretion of bile, which is then stored in the gallbladder. If the liver is taxed or damaged to the extent that bile production is hampered, then the absorption of fat-soluble vitamins and important antioxidants (A, D, E, and K) as well as omega-3s fatty acids will not break down and be absorbed efficiently, or at all, regardless of supplementation methods.

The liver also produces lipoproteins, cholesterol, and phospholipids. In addition, the liver creates GTF (glucose tolerance factor), which acts with insulin to regulate blood sugar levels. Sugars not used as a fuel source are then converted into glycogen in the liver to be stored for future use as an energy source. Moreover, the liver acts to break down critical hormones such as adrenaline, estrogen, insulin, aldosterone. It also as regulates thyroid function (T4 to T3 conversion) which affects weight gain or loss.

In addition to carbohydrate, protein and fat metabolism, the liver functions as a massive remarkable filtering plant for the body, filtering as much as 2 liters of blood per minute. Ammonia, which is toxic to the body, is produced when the amino acids of the protein we consume are broken down (deamination) and mixed with the natural bacteria ripening in the intestines. The liver removes this ammonia along with other metabolic waste products, pharmaceutical drug residue, insecticides ingested with produce, and other chemicals harmful to the human body. It also removes worn out red and white blood cells and bacteria from phagocytosis. In Chinese medicine, the bile is the detergent of the blood.

Eating habits that are problematic for the liver include: the consumption of fried foods, hydrogenated or fractured foods, denatured food products, high saturated fat products and refined sugar products as well as general overeating.

What the liver breaks down is excreted through the kidneys and the bowels. Obviously, regulation of all these organs allows the body to filter and excrete the very poisons that are making us ill. Given past abuses, as well as current pharmaceutical drugs and

OTC (over the counter) drugs an immune suppressed patient may be currently consuming, liver detoxification is essential to good health.

In my clinic I have used several good liver tonification supplements that have been consistently successful in regeneration of the liver. These include: Tumeric Extract (curcuma longa), organic garlic (allium sativum), and Milk Thistle (silybum marianum), which all promote liver protein syntheses. In addition, I supplement methionine, magnesium, Vitamin C, B12 and B5, and folic acid. These supplements are called lipotropic in that they prevent a fatty clogged liver.

These supplements have been used to help people with elevated SGOT and SGPT liver enzyme levels found on your complete blood workup (CBC) performed (hopefully) annually by your doctor. An elevated count of these enzymes suggests that the liver is damaged and shedding its dying cells. Once the supplement routine is implemented for three months, the liver counts usually stabilize to normal.

Detoxification Bath and External Poultices

Since the skin is the body's largest organ, it is only natural that we should detoxify through this passageway. Keeping the skin free of toxins the body has purged, as well as opening the pores to eliminate even more toxins, is a common treatment method across the world. Sweat baths, saunas, even just soaking in the tub for stress, all have been recommended for centuries.

I recommend several ways for my clients to detoxify the skin and the body.

Detoxification Bath: Mix 1 lb. of sea salt with 1 lb. of bicarbonate of soda, add 15 drops of organic chamomile (if allergic to ragweed Do Not use) and soak for 20 minutes. This should be done every change of season at least.

Additionally, hydrotherapy combined with a poultice of tea tree oil, stinging nettle, uva ursi, dandelion and burdock draw out toxins from the liver.

Immune Suppression Detoxification Diet

One of the most important things a severely allergic person suffering from immune suppression or deficiency can do is to continue to follow a detox diet so that their body's energies are not split between fighting their disease and fighting acquired toxins. Even making moderate changes by eliminating several or all of the following mucous and congestion-producing substances - such as baked goods and starch, drugs in general, sweets, refined foods, fried and fatty foods - and by moving toward a more raw and natural diet will encourage detoxification. Diets should be free of artificial sweeteners, irradiated foods, artificial colors, artificial fats, and artificial preservatives. Some examples of detox foods are rice, millet, buckwheat, vegetables (especially squashes), fruits, all green foods (the darker the green the better), herbs and water. One word of caution: be careful of food allergy or sensitivity when choosing foods. Any food can cause sensitivity to the right individual.

It can be difficult to obtain organic and non-artificial food. Most meat sold in supermarkets today (unless otherwise specified as certified organic) contains an enormous amount of antibiotics and steroids due to the inoculation of cattle in the cattle yards. Therefore, abstaining from non-organic meat products can be of enormous help to the constitution of the immunologically compromised person. Meat itself is very difficult to digest in large quantities (over 6 oz.) and even without the chemical additives, can tax the body's energy reserves just in its digestion alone.

Protection from Common Tests Emanating Radiation

Certain foods can protect us and even neutralize the effects from radiation exposure of various western-based tests or treatments. This is critical information for those undergoing X-rays, CAT scans, mammography, radiation therapy and chemotherapy. These low-level radiation methods produce free radicals that can cause damage to lung cells, damage blood vessels, disrupt protein syntheses, alter cell membranes and intracellular structure, and affect DNA and RNA.

The sea vegetable family is premier among foods because sea vegetables are nutrient-packed, can be consumed in the raw state, and are enormously beneficial in pulling off radioactive material. Furthermore, few sea vegetables cause allergic reactions in persons with sensitive immune systems. Sea vegetables contain over 77 minerals and rare earth elements that are in a colloidal form. Colloids are extremely beneficial to the body as they remain in liquid suspension, are very small in size, and are therefore effortlessly absorbed by the body. Sea vegetables containing a nutrient called sodium alginate are especially rich in colloids. Sodium alginate, a complex carbohydrate (polysaccharide) is known for its healing ability. Sodium alginate is highest in concentration in the kelp family, which includes arame, wakame, kombu, hijiki, and of course kelp itself. Moreover, these particular vegetables bind to metal pollutants such as barium, lead, plutonium, cesium, and cadmium and allow for their removal from the human body. These vegetables are also high in vitamin A, all B vitamins, enzymes, and chlorophyll as well as very high in fiber. Another special food that contains a chelation nutrient zybicolinis is unpasteurized miso. Miso is an alkaline-forming fermented soybean paste often eaten as a soup.

Antioxidants and Their Role in Fighting Free Radicals and Cancer

Many people who have asthma are more susceptible to colds, flus and pneumonia due to their use of inhaled steroids or oral steroids (see Chapter 11). Cancer has also been linked to immune suppression. A "cocktail" of the following antioxidants is one of the best insurance policies in the war against immune suppression and its harmful effect on the lungs and skin. I recommend the following forms of traditional antioxidants: for Vitamin A, use natural carotenoids; for Vitamin C, use ester C; for Vitamin E, choose a supplement that includes both tocopherols and tocotrienols. Verify that the supplements are standardized to guarantee their consistent potency. For ease of digestion, choose capsule forms.

Antioxidants

Frequent (every 6 - 8 hours) and daily intake of antioxidants, such as vitamins C and E, grape seed extract and pycnogenol along with many other vitamins, minerals and enzymes, can help asthmatics, especially those with allergies, breathe easier because of their affect on free radicals.

The Department of Environmental Health at the University of Washington in Seattle reported in May of 2000 , "Supplementation of the diet with vitamins E and C benefits asthmatic adults." Nutritionists, bodybuilders and naturopathic doctors have said this for years, but now even modern research says the same thing.

Every day, we hear more and more about free radicals and how they cause damage to our cells and tissues. Overpopulation of these free radicals leads to degeneration of health, the acceleration of the normal aging process and disease. First let's discus what a free radical is. As with many functions of the body, it boils down to chemistry. A free radical is an unstable atom, or group of atoms, that contains one unpaired electron. Since electrons like to hang around in pairs, this electron looks for a mate to stabilize its life and attach itself to. Because the free radical electron bonds so easily, anyone can be its object of affection, with dramatic and costly results.

The free radical family includes superoxides, peroxides, hydroxyls, singlet oxygens, and hypochlorites. Free radicals can make drastic changes in the body's genetic material, destroy cells' protective membranes, cause the cells to hold more water (a part of the aging process) and upset calcium levels in the body all leading to heart disease, cancer and even promote inflammation in the lungs leading to asthma attacks. Once the process of free radical attachment starts, it leads to further production of more free radicals, causing a vicious cycle.

Free radicals are normally prevented from doing any harm by naturally occurring scavengers in the body. These scavengers include SOD (superoxide dismutase), methionine reductase, catalase, and glutathione peroxidase. Ingested nutrients that do this kind of work include Vitamins A, C and E, beta-carotene, selenium, copper, manganese, and the herb bilberry. Additionally, alpha-lipoic acid enhances the antioxidant properties of vitamin A, C and glutathione. [1] These compounds have come to be known as antioxidants. Antioxidants are compounds that protect other compounds from oxidation by being oxidized themselves.

In a study of 17 asthmatics completed by leading author Dr. Carol Trenga, diets were supplemented with daily dosages of 400 IU (international units) of vitamin E, and 500 mg. of vitamin C. The researchers saw an 18% increase in peak flow capacity over those on 'regular' diets, according to the study. More importantly, the authors emphasize that an 18% increase occurred in those asthmatics suffering with the 'most severe' symptoms.

Inflammation that asthmatics have long known about and felt causes high amounts of chronic oxidative stress in the lungs. This oxidative stress needs to be kept in check through proper diet, supplementation, rest and meditation.

Vitamin E

This term usually refers to vitamin E in the form of tocopherols that are comprised of four compounds from plants named alpha, beta, delta, and gamma tocopherol. Vitamin E is a fat-soluble vitamin; it can stay in your body via fat cells. Vitamin E prevents oxidation from happening to fats or lipids and, even more importantly, it can prevent your DNA from mutating. It is especially powerful against oxidation of polyunsaturated fats (a good type of fat), but works on all other types as well. In fact, any cooking or frying of foods will destroy the nutritive properties of vitamin E. When vitamin E attaches to a free radical, it becomes a radical itself — it does not cause damage, but the free radical is deactivated from doing any harm. This vitamin is known to protect the lungs against air pollutants such as nitrogen dioxide and ozone, which can damage the lungs. Vitamin E comes in two forms D, and L; the best kind to take for availability is D-alpha-tocopherol. Vitamin E works best in combination with selenium and Zinc. Selenium and zinc both hold promise as prevention for prostate trouble after age 40.

Vitamin E and Tocotrienol

There is an additional class of vitamin E that also contains alpha, beta, delta and gamma tocotrienols. Several studies have shown that tocotrienols are much stronger than tocopherols with respect to antioxidant, and anticancer properties and cholesterol reduction. Working naturally by reducing the liver's ability to produce cholesterol, tocotrienols, specifically gamma tocotrienol, are valuable in limiting atherosclerosis. In addition to scavenging free radicals, lowering DNA damage, decreasing platelet aggregation, inhibiting inflammation and limiting tumor formations, tocotrienols also penetrate more efficiently into hard to reach areas such as the brain and the liver through its unsaturated side chain.

Vitamin C

Vitamin C has had a long history of recognition. It was discovered almost 3000 years ago, but it was not until the 18th century that it was used on-board ships to prevent scurvy. Researcher Dr. Linus Pauling worked with vitamin C as a super antioxidant. Vitamin C in its pure form is called ascorbic acid and is a water-soluble white powder. Vitamin C seems to be able to reactivate vitamin E so it can be used again to fight free radicals and deactivate them. The human body cannot produce vitamin C.. It is water-soluble and becomes depleted quickly in times of stress; therefore, it does make sense to supplement it. Vitamin C is vital in its work against oxidative damage because it works in some of the most critical areas of defense such as your bloodstream, spinal column, brain and lymphatic fluid, all are watery parts of your body. This includes the liquid on the airway surface part of the lungs. Low vitamin C levels are associated with bronchial tube reactivity.

Some people may have sensitivity to the synthetic vitamin C because it is made from corn sugar. Be careful to consume enough water if you are taking high doses of Vitamin C. High doses of Vitamin C without adequate water intake can cause crystals to form in the kidney and you can end up with kidney stones.

Since vitamin C is an antioxidant, make sure that you are taking a complete array of the other antioxidants as well. Antioxidants work best when taken in combination with one another. Foods lose their antioxidant powers when they are processed and cooked. Stress, air pollution, cigarette smoke and chemicals can cause your body to produce even more free radicals.

B Vitamins

The family of B vitamins is best taken as a team effort, but one or more can be emphasized over the others. Vitamin B1 is synthetically made from wheat. Be careful here if you have allergies to wheat or gluten products. Remember to always take the B-vitamins together (B1, B5, B6, B12 etc.) and since they are water-soluble and get excreted easily, to supplement them 2 - 3x per day in lower amounts (25mg). The Mega B supplements found frequently in health food stores are usually a waste of money because you can only absorb and use so much at time; the rest is urinated right out of the system.

The B vitamins help in everything from nerve communication and red blood cell formation to healthy brain function. They maintain the balance of health in all energy production and help to stabilize the liver. They also maintain healthy sex hormones, mouth, skin, eyes, and hair. It sounds like these vitamins do it all, and they do. The B's need to be taken together, and they all work synergistically, but I would recommend vitamin B3 (niacin) as especially useful for the breakdown and regulation of blood sugar levels. B6 (pyridoxine) and B12 (cyanocobalamin) work well during stressful times, including peak allergic seasons or exposure to toxic environments. Sublingual (under the tongue) B12 is very helpful for my clients who are under a lot of stress.

Supplements

Whole books can be written on the subject of supplements for allergies and asthma. I will give you an overview of what I have found to be useful. Understand that I have never found one supplement alone to be the magic bullet. I do, however, use a shotgun approach; in which each supplement does its tiny part for the greater good of the whole. I have listed quite a few supplements here, some of which has not worked for me, but has reportedly worked for others. Remember: **eat food first, supplement second**.

Another important point to remember is that for gastric juice to be stimulated you need at least 200 calories. What that means is you should take your vitamins with small quantities of food for complete digestion to take place. Remember supplementation is a relatively new invention; prior to that our body's nutrition came from actual food not pills.

In addition to the popular antioxidants (A, E, C), include the following regimen:

Alpha Lipoic Acid

This vitamin has the ability to recycle other antioxidants, such as vitamin C and E and Co-enzyme Q-10, and boost glutathione levels dramatically. Alpha Lipoic Acid exists deep inside every cell of our bodies and works both in fat-soluble and water-soluble body tissues, so it has the greatest range of penetration on the body. It also works in the little furnaces of the body called mitochondria, which affect the body's metabolism by improving waste removal, taking in more nutrients and enhancing the cell's own metabolism and its ability to heal. Alpha Lipoic Acid also has the unique ability to protect patients from the ravages of sugar. Yes, sugar causes immense chemical reactions in the body and Alpha Lipoic Acid helps to absorb the sugar and utilize it more effectively. Think of the implications for diabetics, who already age more rapidly because of the body's inability to control sugar, or for people on prednisone.

NAC N-Acetyl Cysteine

NAC, or N-Acetylcysteine, has in the past been used in liquid form to treat Cystic Fibrosis because it thins mucous secretions. NAC is an antioxidant that stabilizes the free radicals from air pollution. NAC's primary ingredient is a substance called glutathione. Glutathione is thought to repair damage to the lungs, to protect against heavy metals (like lead), and to aid in basic cell metabolism (see glutathione below). NAC reduces lung inflammation from poisons and soothes the lung tissue. It is interesting to note that conventionally, NAC was used to treat liver failure from acetaminophen (Tylenol) poisoning. [2] It has the ability to detoxify some drug overdoses as well as toxic levels of metals in the body.

L-Glutathione

Glutathione is a protein produced in the liver that is in most cells of the body. Glutathione assists in amino acid transport mechanisms and assists in the treatment of blood and liver disorders. It also protects cells from oxidative stress, (a cause of aging), heavy metal toxicity and prevents free radical pathology. In HIV research, glutathione has been shown to block the signaling of the binding site that normally initiates virus replication. It has also been shown in research to reduce the side effects of adriamycin, a very powerful chemotherapy drug. Glutathione also protects cells from cigarette smoke, exposure to radiation (x-rays) and alcohol.

Melatonin

Melatonin is a hormone that is a powerful scavenger of the hydroxyl radical, one of the most lethal free radicals made by the body. Supplementation may be necessary, especially in older patients who may have lower levels of melatonin because the pineal gland lowers its production as one ages. Caution: do not mix NSAIDS with melatonin.

Green Tea

(camellia sinensis) extract with at least 75% polyphenols

There is a difference between the black tea I grew up with and green tea. Black tea is left to darken and oxidize for many hours after it has been harvested; where as green tea is packaged right away. Green tea contains polyphenolic compounds called epicatechins that possess antiinflammatory actions as well as anticarcinogenic properties and aid in detoxification. In addition, it prevents oxidation of LDL cholesterol and raises "good" HDL cholesterol. Moreover, it produces good bacteria in the intestinal tract (Lactobacilli and Bififobacteria) while suppressing the bad (such as Enterobacteriaceae) and at the same time kills cavity-causing bacteria and reduces plaque in the mouth.

Green tea in particular contains many different compounds, as there are many different kinds of green tea. One of the most prevalent compounds is catechin, which has antioxidant properties. It reduces the clotting tendency of the blood, strengthens the resistance of capillaries, and lowers cholesterol. From ancient times until the nineteenth century, it was used to prevent tooth decay. The Chinese have used tea as therapy for 4,000 years, recent studies have shown that green tea can be used as a method of thermogenesis, or fat burning. It has also been shown to have stress-reducing and antianxiety effects without the sedating effects of other agents or drugs. In a Japanese study, one of green teas key ingredients, L-theanine, has been shown to support healthy blood pressure, enhance concentration and learning, promote mental clarity and enhance immune function. Only one word of caution: excessive amounts of tea (as well as coffee, calcium, zinc or manganese) can all inhibit iron absorption.

Grape Seed Extract

Much like pycogenol, grape seed extract is a powerful protector against oxidative damage, but I find clients have less allergic sensitivity to the grape seed extract. Perhaps this is because people can be sensitive to pine bark. Grapes seem to be low on the allergic list. Choose a grape seed extract that contains at least 85% of proanthocyanidins.

Rooibos Tea

Rooibos is a red tea from South Africa that is marvelous in taste and extremely satisfying. Unlike other teas and coffee, Rooibos tea contains few tannins or tannic acid, the main culprit in iron loss in the body. Studied heavily in Japan, Rooibos has been shown to reduce insomnia, mild depression, stomach cramps, colic, constipation, and most importantly to us, allergic symptoms including itching and skin irritations.

Rooibos contains an element called alpha-hydroxy acid which promotes healthy skin, along with the minerals iron, potassium, zinc, magnesium, fluoride and manganese. High in antioxidants, including vitamin E, C, bioflavonoids and carotene, this tea was able to inhibit cancer-causing effects of x-rays in animal studies! It also contains flavonoids (specifically aspalathin) that have been demonstrated to reduce leg cramps and alleviate skin and circulation problems. It also contains SOD, an enzyme that protects against oxidative stress by scavenging free radicals and reducing inflammation.

Photochemicals: Their Food Sources and Actions

I have provided on the next page a list of plant-based foods, the substances found in them that are essential to health, called "photochemicals" (from photosynthesis) and their effects of these photochemicals on the human body[1].

Photochemicals: Their food sources and actions

Food Source	Name	Action in the body
Deeply pigments fruits and vegetables (carrots, sweet potatoes, tomatoes, spinach, broccoli, cantaloupe, pumpkin, apricots)	Carotenoids (including beta-carotene)	Act as anti-oxidants, reducing the risk of cancer
Citrus fruits	Limonene	Triggers enzyme production to facilitate carcinogen excretion
	Phenols	Inhibit lipid oxidation, block formation of carcinogenic nitrosamines in the body
Garlic/onions	Allyl sulfides	Trigger enzyme production to facilitate carcinogen excretion
Broccoli and other cruciferous vegetables (cauliflower and brussels sprouts)	Sulforaphane Dithiolthiones	Protects against cancer Trigger enzyme production to block carcinogenic damage to cells DNA
	Indoles	Trigger enzymes to inhibit estrogen action, reducing the risk of breast cancer
	Isothiocyanates	Trigger enzyme production to block carcinogenic damage of cell's DNA
Grapes	Ellagic Acid	Scavenges carcinogens
Flaxseed	Lignans	Block estrogen activity in cells, reducing the risk of breast and ovarian cancer
Soy/legumes	Protease inhibitors	Suppress enzyme production in cancer cells, slowing tumor growth Inhibit cell reproduction in the GI tract, preventing colon cancer
	Phytosterols	Block estrogen activity in cells, reducing the risk of breast and ovarian cancer
	Isoflaveniods	Block estrogen activity in cells, reducing the risk of breast and ovarian cancer
	Saponins	Interfere with DNA reproduction, preventing cancer cell multiplication
Fruits (blueberries, prunes, grapes), oats, soybeans	Caffeic acid	Triggers enzyme production to make carcinogens water soluble, facilitating excretion
	Ferulic acid	Binds to nitrates in stomach, preventing conversion to nitrosamines
Grains	Phylic acid	Binds to minerals, preventing cancer causing free radical formation
Fruits, vegetables, tea, wine, oregano	Flavonoids	Act as anti-oxidants, reducing the risk of cancer

Ginger

There are two types of ginger: aged ginger called "mother" ginger and fresh ginger called "baby" ginger. For cooking, fresh ginger is typically used. For therapeutic purposes, as a Yang restorative for example, "mother" ginger (gan jiang) is typically used to stimulate the Lungs and Spleen. It reduces phlegm in the body, stimulates circulation and increases peristalsis in the colon. One of the interesting properties of ginger, from the Chinese perspective, is that it helps relieve invasion of the Wei chi fields, your first line of immune defense.

Litchi (Lychee)

Litchi works as an energy stimulant and affects the Spleen and the Liver. Eat the steamed and dried litchis as an alternative means of controlling asthma. I have never personally tried this method, but I am sure I will in the future. According to Traditional Chinese Medicine (TCM) it promotes the production of body fluids and helps replenish injured Blood.

Pumpkin

Fresh pumpkin contains B vitamins, protein, essential fatty acids and Zinc, all substances usually deficient in people with allergies. Use approximately one pound of fresh-steamed pumpkin mixed with honey as a daily therapy.

Phosphatidylserine

Phosphatidylserine is a newly packaged supplement used to treat adrenocortical dysfunction (adrenal burnout). It is also used for delaying the decline of neurotransmitter function associated with the aging process and is touted an anti-aging supplement, especially for memory. It is well known for repairing damage done by excessive stress hormone release. It has the ability to regulate cortisol within the body, especially if one has high cortisol levels. Clinical tests using computer and performance (neuropsychological) tests showed improvements in sleep and mental function. Phosphatidylserine is a major component of brain cell membranes and its production drops with age. Usually it is manufactured from soybeans, so be cautious if you have any soy sensitivity.

Forskolin

Forskolin has been found to stimulate release of thyroid hormone thereby relieving symptoms of hypothyroidism such as fatigue, depression, weight gain, and dry skin. Forskolin is a powerful activator of the enzyme adenylcyclase, which increases the signal carrier cyclic AMP in cells. Low amounts of cyclic AMP have been found to be associated with asthma, heart disease, high blood pressure, glaucoma, eczema, and psoriasis. WARNING: Forskolin relaxes the bronchial muscles and may dangerously increase the potency of certain asthma medications such as Albuterol, theophylline, and beclomethasone. If you have low blood pressure or duodenal ulcers, consult a doctor or naturopath before consumption.

Localized Honey

Honey is an enormously valuable food that can sustain life and has for almost 8,000 years. It is listed as a food and medicine in many ancient books, such as the Old and New Testaments of the Bible, the Koran, and several Taoist medical books in China. Hippocrates cured skin disorders with honey. Honey's wound healing ability has been documented by modern research methods as early as the 1930's. It has been used around the world for healing of burns, wounds, and infections.

Usually the darker the honey the higher the antioxidants in it. Research shows that many bacteria that cause such diseases as Cholera, Meningitis, Pneumonia, Septicemia, urinary infections, and even anthrax are vulnerable to the antimicrobial activity of honey. A special strain of honey called manuka honey has shown to be effective in treating the Helicobacter Pylori bacteria responsible for peptic ulcers and some forms of cancer. Mostly I use honey for its anti-inflammatory properties.

I try to use localized honey as an immunity booster. Because the bees gather honey from the local plants and flowers, it acts when ingested as a mild inoculation of environmental factors that you may be allergic to as a whole such as tree, bush and crop pollens that can affect you in the growing season (seasonal allergies). Do not overdose initially; gradually build up your immunity as more is not necessarily better. I have found for myself, that bee pollen and bee propolis are too strong for my system, but they may be all right with yours.

Throughout the day I will frequently mix honey and a fresh lemon slice in a glass of room temperature water to sustain my energy, to prevent brain fog, and to control my weight from excess snacking.

Pycnogenol

Pycnogenol is a natural plant extract made from the bark of the Maritime Pine tree growing on the coast of France. When referring to pycnogenol, most people are referring to oligomeric proanthocyanidins (OPCs), which are flavonols that are powerful antioxidants and have excellent bioavailability. Clinical tests show that as an antioxident, OPC may be as much as fifty times more potent than vitamin E and twenty times more potent as vitamin C!

Pycnogenol contains approximately 40 natural ingredients, including proanthocyanidins, a special class of bioflavonoids, organic acids and other biologically active components. It also contains water-soluble organic acids, organic acid glusides and glucose esters, as well as other highly useful biologically active compounds

For asthmatics and people with eczema or dermatitis, Pycnogenol improves circulation and skin smoothness, fights inflammation, and strengthens the circulatory system.

Pycnogenol also readily binds to collagen fibers, thus improving the elasticity and integrity of connective tissues. These attributes and more make Pycnogenol a prime protector against the effects of early aging and even against the far-reaching effects of prednisone.

Quercetin

Quercetin is a bioflavonoid (sometimes referred to as vitamin P) which the body cannot synthesize, so it must be obtained from food or supplementation. The most important thing that bioflavonoids do is strengthen the capillary beds in conjunction with vitamin C; in this way they can help with the bumps and bruises of everyday living. Quercetin is found in blue-green algae from the ocean and has been used successfully in the prevention of asthma breathlessness. Short of consuming some of the "Green Drinks" out there, quercetin probably is best acquired from supplement form.

Shark Liver Oil or Alkylglycerol

Alkylglycerol or AKG is a group of compounds that help in the production and/or stimulation of white blood cells, specifically, the macrophages which help consume viruses. The highest concentration of AKGs comes from the liver of the deep-water shark. Shark liver oil, especially of the Greenland shark, has been shown a valuable antioxidant. According to Dr. Ingemar Joelsson, the AKGs in shark liver oil are unique in that they attack and eliminate free radicals that have penetrated the cell wall. Most antioxidants that we know of are only effective in scavenging free radicals outside the cell wall. Most importantly, the supplement appears to be safe without any significant side effects. [3]

Borage Seed Oil

Of all supplements that I take, Borage seed oil is a wonderful supplement for those who have dry itchy skin. It has made the most notable difference in my skin. Its primary ingredient is gamma linolenic acid (GLA), which soothes and moisturizes the skin from the inside out. GLA works as a natural antiinflammatory, but also purges arachidonic acid from the body. When arachidonic acid accumulates in the body, pain and inflammation are the result. Natural sources of this product include nuts, seeds and grains. Actually, the richest source available is mothers' milk. Spirulina is a very rich source of GLA in the plant world, however, and may be easier to obtain. GLAs also strengthen immunity and inhibit excessive cell division (cancer).

In the supplement line, there are three other choices of getting your GLA's: Borage seed oil, Evening primrose oil, and black currant seed oil. I like the supplement of Borage seed oil. Borage seed oil is the richest source containing about 20 to 23 percent of GLA. Evening primrose oil contains about 8 to 10 percent, and Black current seed oil contains about 15 to 17 percent GLA as well as 10 to 12 percent of alpha-linolenic acid an omega-3 oil. Make sure that you buy oils manufactured with a cold pressed extraction process, which yields a much cleaner product. Solvent extraction is a cheaper method, but may lead to degradation and contamination.

When dealing with an acute attack of eczema or dermatitis, I initially use a loading dose. A 1300mg capsule generally contains about 312 mg. of GLA. Take as many as eight capsules a day for about two weeks and then gradually cut back to only one or two a day, depending on your body-weight. If you begin to get diarrhea, then obviously cut back to a lower dosage. Maintenance doses of 150 mg. GLA are appropriate for vegetarians; if you eat meat, you probably need more than 150 mg., but no more than 350 mg.

Zinc

Zinc is a wonder vitamin that is usually lacking in the diet of immune system sufferers. Zinc is itself an antioxidant; it protects the liver from chemical damage stemming from preservatives and prescription drugs, it helps to form bone and to produce collagen. It helps the blood use vitamin E and assists in the absorption of vitamin A. Good sources are sardines, brewers yeast, kelp, fish in general, and pecans. In addition, I use a sublingual Zinc for more efficient absorption.

Magnesium

Magnesium deficiency can make every disease worse because magnesium is involved in controlling nerve and muscle impulses in the body as well as helping to assist in pH regulation. It is vital that asthmatics, sufferers of chronic fatigue syndrome (CFS), irritable bowel syndrome (IBS), depression, hypertension, and anyone with heart ailments have their magnesium levels monitored because magnesium affects all energy production in the body.

In addition magnesium prevents the calcification of soft tissue and bone. Good sources are dairy, fish, meat and seafood. Spinach, chocolate, tea and almonds can interfere with its absorption.

Violence and Supplementation

In relation to supplements and children, a rigorously monitored study competed by Oxford University in Britain involving youthful offenders and vitamin supplementation showed the true benefits and power of this simple therapy. Some youthful offenders were given adequate amounts of vitamins, mineral and essential fatty acids, while other convicts in a control group were given a placebo. Researchers then recorded the number of disciplinary actions taken against these inmates. The results were astounding: there was a 35.1 percent reduction in offenses in the treatment group, while the placebo group showed no reduction. The Oxford researchers concluded that "antisocial behaviors in prisons, including violence are reduced by vitamins, mineral and essential fatty acids." They also suggested "similar implications for those eating poor diets in the community". The final line is that violence and misbehavior could be reduced at the cost of $1.50 per day!

Miscellaneous

I also use herbals in the maintenance of allergies including: wild yam, milk thistle, cayenne, and alfalfa. A naturopathic doctor or herbalist can help you decide if any of these would be right for you.

(1) *Prescription for Nutritional Healing; James F. Balch*
(2) *The Nutraceutical Revolution, Richard Firshein, Page 191-2.*
(3) *Shark Liver Oil Nature's Amazing Healer, Neil Solomon, MD PhD., Richard Passwater. PhD., Ingemar Johnson MD, PhD., Kensington Health 1997*

CHAPTER 7

Exercise

"You cannot get wet with the word water"

-Alan Watts

I think I am one of the odd ones in the world today. I actually like to exercise. I like all forms of exercise, from walking to skiing to martial arts, right back to lifting weights. I enjoy sweating. I like the burn that happens in my muscles when I have used them extensively. I feel exhilarated after a workout and I look forward to the next one.

All right, I will quit rambling on about how wonderful exercise is. The fact is, if you are an asthmatic you may have hated any form of exercise in the past because it may have caused you to wheeze, or worse. Getting asthmatics to exercise and be active sometimes can be a challenge. I have worked with the local American Lung Association and the American Respiratory Alliance for many years. We have frequent summer asthma camps called "Camp Breathe E-Z" for children age five and up. Even at this young age, some children are apprehensive to exercise, even if it is fun.

The truth is that the United States is in trouble with overweight and obese men, women and children. The National Institutes of Health state that over one-half of the population is overweight! Worse than that, 20% of the population will die prematurely due to obesity! One reason may be that only 22% of the population exercises five times a week for more than 30 minutes. As I type on my computer I think of this fact: All things being equal, if I were to change back from typing on my computer to using an old manual typewriter, I would lose 10 pounds in one year just from that one change of effort! The truth is we don't move around like we used to.

My love affair with exercise started when I was about eight years old. I had been reading about exercise programs and the lifestyle of many famous strongmen. Back then exercise was called "physical culture." Of course, being healthy like the men in the magazines was a fantasy for me. Thanks in part to my frequent asthma attacks and to the drug prednisone, I was very physically weak, I had no endurance, and very little muscle tone.

I hated being this weak and so very vulnerable. Whether the game was baseball, football or horseshoes, the smallest kids, even those younger than I, could out throw me. They could out run me in sprints - forget about me even trying a long 100-yard dash! I had no physical strength at all and wrestling around was out of the question. Even though I was taking Judo lessons from a very patient martial arts instructor, I decided that I would have to do something to help myself. I prayed to God nightly to help me, but every morning I would wake up and no muscles had grown.

Judo training was very important to me at that time in my life. Judo allowed me as an individual to do something as an individual at my own pace, but I could still compete and be in a sport. My Judo instructor was excellent at pushing me, but not too hard. I grew to love the philosophy of the East and the martial arts, especially the mental focus and discipline that martial arts provides as well as the honor and respect that tradition teaches. These are important for all children, not just to asthmatics.

Please understand at this point in time (1967-68) there were neither asthma nor severe allergy medications to speak of. Benadryl was a prescription drug! My parents had tried every pediatrician in the area and even out of our state. We even tried alternative methods recommended at that time by physicians. Nothing worked. All we could do was treat some of the symptoms.

I finally talked to my parents about praying to God for help to make me strong and about what to do to help myself. My father is a very devout Catholic, and he did not want me to stop praying. His enlightened words are something he and my mother would repeat to me often when I was discouraged, down, and feeling beaten. "God helps those who help themselves," Mom and Dad would say. How profound. What an awakening I had. I no longer was going to wait for God to bestow a miracle on me. I no longer was waiting for the doctor to give me a shot and cure me. I no longer was counting on someone else to make me better. I understood that healing of any sort has to begin from your own heart, your own intentions, and your own effort.

I understood at age eight what so many people I later encountered–as a personal trainer did not understand as adults. Life is tough for many of us, regardless of what ailments or diseases you might have. It sometimes takes work just to get through the day with a good attitude and not have it ruined by a simple event that takes seconds.

If you are to survive, you have to get tough, get aggressive and get in control. This is especially true if you have any affliction going on in your life. You cannot expect someone else to heal you, including your parents, spouse or any one else who loves you that deeply. YOU must be the one in charge. It is your responsibility to have the fight, the drive to succeed, and the tenacity to bring your commitment to health to fruition.

All that being said, you also need a good support network of people who truly love and nurture you in order to heal as well as good coaches or teachers. We are all human, and we all stumble and even fall backwards sometimes. These people are here to dust you off, encourage you again, and help you on your journey. Notice I did not say anything about someone picking you up when you fall. You must do that yourself. You must have the will to get up yourself. Otherwise, all the encouragement in the world will only serve as a temporary save.

Good teachers and coaches help to point you in the right direction, to open your mind, and to expose you to options that you perhaps have not thought of. Even the word doctor originates from the Latin word teacher. My parents and my Judo instructor were my teachers and I was determined to teach or doctor myself into being well.

So I decided to make myself strong, to regenerate this weak and frail body of mine that was sensitive to everything. I started doing push-ups and sit-ups. I began lifting my legs to my chest in rapid succession. I did jumping jacks, burpees, and isometric exercises. I read all I could on the subject of exercise. Bruce Lee fascinated me because he was such a proponent of exercise and training. I read karate books, boxing books and even wrestling books. One of the best books I ever read was the Boxer's Training book by the Ring. It had so many interesting exercises that boxers used to train. I began to train as the boxers did. One of the favorite exercises for boxers in the days of Rocky Graciano was to cut wood with an axe. I asked my Dad to let me have an axe so I could cut wood and exercise. He just smiled and said, "we have 14 acres of woods to cut, help yourself".. Every winter (because of too much pollen in the spring and summer) I would cut wood for whomever wanted it for their fireplace.

I begged my parents for a chest expander cable set and a pair of handgrips for Christmas. I had read that a chest expander was a surefire way to add muscles to your frame regardless of how skinny you were. Even back before the day of infomercials and the Internet, I was influenced by good marketing techniques. Christmas morning I woke up, and like magic, the chest expander was underneath the tree. I was so excited! Now I could be built like the guys in the magazines with just a few workouts a week!

I used the chest expanders faithfully every morning before school. Pretty soon, I had worked my way from being able to pull only one spring, to three springs, and then four. I was making progress, but I wanted more. For my birthday, I asked for a 110 pound steel barbell set. Now this was the way to gain strength I thought. In my mind, only the real strongmen used barbells, and I was finally strong enough to use the weights.

I also continued my martial arts training everyday. In addition to cutting wood, I stretched my muscles and tendons, practiced my kicks, punches and blocks, hit the heavy bag and settled in for at least a half hour to an hour of meditation everyday. This was my ritual day after day, year after year. This was my life choice that commanded me to become the best I could be.

I scoured the magazines and books for routines that I was to follow in order to become the strongman of my dreams. I read exercise physiology textbooks and studied Grays Anatomy. I was determined to be strong and have some muscle to my body. I found several routines that probably had been forgotten with time. I continue to workout to this day, although my body is built more like that of a strongman on ESPN than of a bodybuilder or movie star, it is all natural (I never took anabolic steroids). Sometimes building a body that is truly functional and strong is more important than aesthetics. I maintain functional strength that most people are surprised at to this day, in spite of long bouts of muscle-depleting prednisone.

Now we have Nautilus, Keaiser, Hammer Strength, and every other manufacturer of strength and exercise training equipment, and I will share with you some of the best basic exercises for asthmatics to perform.

The most important thing that exercise can do for you is to physically change your body's chemistry. We have all heard of stories- and maybe you even know someone -who was told by their doctor "start exercising and you won't have to go on blood pressure medication or cholesterol medication or diabetic medication." What they are essentially telling you is that with consistency and the right program, exercise will change your blood chemistry and your pH levels in as little as three months! Many people fail to realize that hard, vigorous exercise is what keeps people young. By age 40, everyone slows down, some people to a crawl, but this is the time that exercise is most important.

Cardiovascular Vs. Fat Burning Differences

In this section I will describe, with great injustice to exercise physiology, the difference between fat burning exercise and cardiovascular exercise.

Workouts are like investing your money. We want a guaranteed return for our investment with minimal risk. We also demand that there be tangible results we can see. If a mutual fund prospectus were to project a loss of income over the next 10 years, we would abandon that particular fund and move our money somewhere else. Exercise programs are similar in our expectations.

Let us look at fat burning first, since most people have at least a mild interest in doing that. As an asthmatic myself, I understood that being overweight was a strain on my heart and my lungs. My body had to labor so much more intensely to move me around if I were heavy. I read once that for every pound you are overweight, you can subtract one month of life from your longevity. For every 60 minutes you exercise per day, you can add a day to your life.

The body is constructed to store fat as a self-preservation mechanism. Not only does fat allow us to have an indefinite supply of fuel, but it also protects the body with padding (fat), if you will. The food we eat, if not consumed by activity, repair, or basal metabolism, is stored for future use as fat. It does not matter if the food is carbohydrate, protein or fat in nature. If fuel is not used, it is stored. This is a simple fact that will never change in the evolution of a human being. No diet, supplement, drug, special technique, or anything else will change this fact, although the superior marketing techniques of many retail companies may tempt us to believe otherwise.

Our bloodstream carries oxygen to various cells in our body, which mixes with the fuel (stored food) to create energy for all sorts of tasks. The food is the fuel and the oxygen is the spark that ignites the fuel to burn as calories. The more intense the activity or demand for fuel, the greater the oxygen demand to strike the match. This is called aerobic metabolism.

For sport and health, athletes include in their training programs workouts for strength training, anaerobic and aerobic conditioning. The heart muscle is a muscle, like the muscle in your leg or arm, but is composed of a different kind of muscle tissue. All forms of training (strength training, anaerobic and aerobic conditioning) have been shown to assist the heart muscle in becoming stronger. Through training, the heart grows stronger and more efficient at pumping oxygen-rich-blood to your body tissues. Through training we can take a heart that normally beats at 75 times per minute down to 55 times per minute which is quite a difference in labor for a small muscle the size of your fist! This is one of the greatest ways to increase longevity and health regardless of your age.

The heart is an amazing organ. During peak effort, your heart rate may increase two to three times its normal resting rate! During exercise testing to determine maximum heart rates on treadmills and stationary bikes, the treadmill produced higher heart rate values. Later I will outline a treadmill training programs just for asthmatics. Children also have a higher maximal heart rate than adults do. Their heart rate can be driven up to 215 beats per minute! Once matured, their maximum heart rate drops with age to a rate of 0.7 to 0.8 beat per minute for every year they get older regardless of sex, level of conditioning, or environment!

To burn fat and a maximum number of calories we must maintain a target heart rate of at least 70 to 75% of our maximum for at least 20 minutes. We must also use large muscle groups, such as the entire leg, buttocks and upper back, and do this in a continuous fashion for at least 15 minutes.

There is a law of diminishing returns for your fat-burning workouts. Approximately 45-minutes into your exercise program, the body starts to lessen its rapid consumption of calories, and begins to slow down its fuel burning process in an effort to conserve the fat reserves of the body. This template means that your fat-burning workouts should not exceed 45 minutes. You would be better served doing two, 20 to 25 minutes workouts per day than one long hour workout! That little fact is the tried and true secret to managing the time invested in exercise to the greatest result.

Cardiovascular workouts, on the other hand, train the heart to work at a level closer to the maximum heart rate that you can sustain. The workout itself may take you up to 85 to 95% of your maximum heart rate (Obviously, if you have heart disease, this is not a good thing to do without a physician's supervision). At this point, however, the body no longer is burning fat as its fuel source, but is burning carbohydrate (blood sugar, liver sugar) because carbohydrate is much quicker to convert to fuel as your intensity increases. The more intense the exercise, the more carbohydrate (sugar) you burn. Here is the breakdown on fuel sources used by the body.

Technically speaking, all percentages are based on VO2 max or the maximum oxygen consumption and your maximum heart rate. So, for example, if you are using 40% of your maximum allowable heart beats per minute, then you are using fat stores as the major fuel source to move the body. The actual breakdown is:

Less than 40% the body uses all fat for fuel

40% to 75% the body uses a mix of fat and carbohydrate for fuel

75% to 80% the body uses mostly carbohydrate for fuel

80% the body uses all carbohydrate for fuel

For asthmatics, the body's ability to process and deliver clean oxygen may be the limiting factor. Many times, it is difficult to train because we cannot get the same amount of fresh oxygen per breath as a normal person. This limit can be offset by the breathing, meditation and stress management techniques I will describe later in this book. (Information on purchasing my CD and videotapes on meditation, stress management and QiGong techniques is located in the back of this book.)

Training is even more important for the asthmatic than for athletes because we need to make our hearts more efficient in their functioning. The heart has to be strong to survive the stress of having an asthma attack. Since the heart is the pump that pushes the oxygen rich-blood to the tissues, when we do not get the oxygen we need, the poor heart labors intensely to push more blood through to nourish the starving tissues. No wonder we are so tired after a prolonged asthma attack; we have just run a marathon!

Before Starting an Exercise Program

It's always a good idea to have your physician's blessing before starting an exercise program.......

If you haven't been exercising, you need to take this slowly, trying a few repetitions of each exercise. Remember set your goals based on your abilities ...not anyone else's.

Water

I cannot stress enough the importance of drinking plenty of clean, filtered, treated water. The reason I suggest drinking treated water because one study by the EPA stated that many cities had over seven hundred chemicals suspended in their drinking water supplies, including lead. [1] In one study completed by the Virginia Dept. of Health, 58% of individual wells tested were contaminated with coliform bacteria.

Whether you live on a farm and have well water or use the city water out of the tap, have the water tested regularly for contaminants. If there are more than 10,000 people using your water system, get a copy of your Consumer Confidence Report (CCR). This report will tell you where your water comes from and whether or not it exceeds EPA limits of over 80 plus different chemicals.

If you have well water, make sure that it is tested every couple of years. Your filtration system should be based on what your test results report is in your water. A nonprofit group called National Sanitation Foundation (NSF) tests and certifies home water treatment systems. The NSF seal also certifies that the home filtration system you buy does what it says it will do. Check out their web site at www.nsf.org for more information.

Air Passages: Exercise

Two contaminants that can be especially deadly for asthmatic children are nitrates and nitrites. These can cause a sometimes-fatal condition in which the hemoglobin in the blood is reduced. Hemoglobin carries oxygen in the blood stream. These contaminants have also been associated with stomach cancers.

There is no guarantee that chlorinated water is microbe-free. In testing, some microbes, like E-coli, are used as an indicator bacteria that accurately predict the presence of other pathogens. Some pathogens, like cryptosporidium, are not totally eliminated by chlorination either.

The ideal water treatment system is a combination of several systems. I recommend filtering in multiple stages. First, a series of canister prefilters take out the dirt, chlorine and ground contaminants in descending order of 25, then 15 , and finally down to .05 microns. Next, use an activated carbon filter system and finally run the filtered water through a UV light attached to the water line. All of these filters should be in place prior to water entering your hot water tank or any other water line in your house.

I like the reverse osmosis system because it removes dissolved solids (like lead), bacteria, hydrocarbons, asbestos, viruses, most pesticides and other chemicals. Reverse osmosis does not remove chloroform, but adding an activated carbon filter will take care of that, as well as bad tastes and odors. The only problem with reverse osmosis water system is that it takes all the minerals out of the water and when consumed, the water can actually leech the minerals from the human body. If you use this method make sure that you add minerals back into your diet or possibly back into the water system itself.

A note here on UV light systems for killing bacteria. Usually they are about 80% effective when they start, but lose their effectiveness as they age, so change the UV bulbs often.

Drink at least 16 ounces of water one hour before you get on your treadmill and begin your warmup. One big gulp of water usually equals about an ounce. I find that room temperature water is less of a shock on my lungs, since the body does not have to warm it to core temperature. This is especially true if you are the type of asthmatic who reacts negatively to cold air or a sudden change in temperature. Remember, the whole idea is to train to your utmost tolerance/capacity. By warming up and drinking fluids, you are enhancing the probability of having a productive workout.

Right before your workout, drink another 6 ounces of room temperature water. While drinking your water, set a realistic goal for what you are going to do that day. Is it a good day, or have you been wheezing all night? Common sense really applies here. If you are having a bad day, you may just want to cut the workout time in half and continue with the warmup through the duration of the time you decided on. I always did my workouts regardless of how I felt. That was me. I figured a little bit of movement could only help me. Most times by lying around, not moving the blood, and not allowing the core temperature to rise up results in thickening the mucous more.

During the actual workout itself, drink 4 to 6 ounces of water every 10 to 15 minutes! For every pound you lose during your exercise routine, replace it with 16 ounces of water. Not soda, not fruit juice, and definitely not alcohol! Water is what makes your cells work optimally. The cells are made of 70% water, not cola or apple juice. Not only do the cells in your lungs need to remove waste products, but so do the cells in your heart, muscles and everywhere else in your body. Give the body the tools it needs to function correctly.

Warm up First - ALWAYS!

The more severe your asthma is, the more gradually you have to ease into exercise. If you have asthma give yourself at least 12 - 15 minutes to warm up at an extremely easy pace. The warmup allows your diaphragm to become prepared for heavier breathing and will prevent the common "stitch" or pain in the side that we hear about frequently.

How do you warm up? Take 12 to 20 minutes and exercise lightly on the treadmill, the bike or with light calisthenics. Even marching in place will work, so don't let lack of equipment be an excuse. Personally, I think it makes more sense to imitate as closely as possible in warmup the actual exercise you want to perform. In other words, if you are going to be doing weighted squats as a part of your exercise program, a portion of your warmup should be squatting a few times with just your body weight.

Treadmill

For asthmatics young or old, one of the best investments is a treadmill for cardiovascular health and overall fat burning. Having a treadmill in your home is the ideal way to control your exercise environment. Of course controlling your environment is crucial to asthmatics and people with allergies. Like no other environment, you have the most control over dust, dust mites, perfumes, pollen, and all other asthma-triggers in your home. It is your sanctuary. At home you also have the convenience of being able to workout whenever you are at your best, you have the ability to measure exact distance and your speed, you can calibrate your progress accurately on machines that let you store your personal best times and distances, and you are never too far from the kids.

For some people like me, the best exercise time is mid afternoon. That may not work for some people, and they may do better in the morning or evening. Not only do you have to weigh your asthma factors, but your energy level as well. Some people just will never be morning people, let alone get up before work or school to exercise! Many people just do not have the time during the day (you can only get up so early) and may have to exercise at night. Exercise when you can, that is better than no exercise at all!

A Treadmill Program for Asthmatics

Please remember that to be effective in your exercise program, you must train smart. For asthmatics, training smart means warming up at least 3 times longer than for non-asthmatics. This even applies to walking for distance. For example, if you can walk comfortably for a distance of 1 to 2 miles at 2.5 miles per hour, then warm up at 2.0 m.p.h. for 3 minutes, 2.2 or 2.3 m.p.h. for 3 minutes, and then gradually inch it up .1 m.p.h. every 2 minutes until you hit 12 minutes total. Then you can start training. For some, walking 1 to 2 miles may be a lot. Regardless, the 12-minute warmup will allow ample time for your blood to thin, warm, and dilate your capillaries. For many asthmatics, any sudden burst of activity really flares their lungs into spasm.

After you warmup, begin training at a little higher level of intensity, but not too quickly. Say you can walk comfortably at 2.5 m.p.h. for 30 minutes. This rate and time has no adverse affect on your asthma and is easy, even though you may break a sweat towards the end. Move the speed up to 2.6 or 2.7 and see if you can walk for 30 minutes without any adverse affect again. If this speed is okay, maintain that speed/time for a week or so. Than move it a notch again, say to 2.8 or 2.9 for 30 minutes. Continue to do this until you reach your maximum walking speed. I have found that most people have trouble walking any faster than 4.5 m.p.h. for 30 minutes regardless of their physical condition (asthma or not). This is just a benchmark to go on. It has to do more with leg stride than actual fitness, as most people try to jog after this point. Someone with long legs will be able to go much faster and someone who is 5 feet tall may have to go slower. Realize this and adapt based on your own physiology.

One of the greatest hints I can offer you as an asthmatic and as a personal trainer is to do a little every day rather than too much in several days. You will reap more benefit, for example, by walking on the treadmill every day for 20 minutes in the afternoon 6 days a week, than doing two, 1-hour workouts twice a week! More is not necessarily better! This is true not only for asthmatics trying to increase their breathing and endurance capacity, but also for people trying to burn fat and lose weight. If you are trying to do both, boy is this the program for you!

After you can walk for 30 minutes at your maximum walking speed, where you feel like you need to start jogging, begin a run/walk program.

Walk/Jog Program

All asthmatics will find their own unique mannerisms with their body. Some will have to warm up more than 12 - 15 minutes to get the desired result of exercise without bronchial spasm. Learn to become your own best doctor and err on the side of conservatism.

Try to work out in a place that is cleaned regularly, and to avoid dust, that does not have a carpet on the floor as carpets can hold dust. The room should be well ventilated, and the air should move around slightly. The humidity should be less than 60% and the drier the better. The room temperature should not exceed 72 degrees F, with 70 degrees or below being more comfortable to exercise in.

Air Passages: Exercise

First do a warmup for 12 - 15 minutes and then stretch. Then do the walk/jog program below. At the end of the workout, stretch again.

Week 1	Walk 5 minutes, jog 1 minute, walk 5 minutes. Repeat 4 times.
Week 2	Walk 5 minutes, jog 2 minutes, walk 5 minutes. Repeat 4 times.
Week 3	Walk 5 minutes, jog 3 minutes, walk 4 minutes. Repeat 4 times.
Week 4	Walk 5 minutes, jog 4 minutes, walk 3 minutes. Repeat 4 times.
Week 5	Walk 5 minutes, jog 4 minutes, walk 3 minutes. Repeat 4 times.
Week 6	Walk 5 minutes, jog 5 minutes, walk 3 minutes. Repeat 3 times.
Week 7	Walk 5 minutes, jog 7 minutes, walk 5 minutes. Repeat 2 times.
Week 8	Walk 5 minutes, jog 7 minutes, walk 3 minutes. Repeat 3 times.
Week 9	Walk 5 minutes, jog 10 minutes, walk 5 minutes. Repeat 2 times.
Week 10	walk 5 minutes, jog 10 minutes, walk 2 minutes. Repeat 2 times.
Week 11	Walk 5 minutes, jog 12 minutes, walk 4 minutes. Repeat 2 times.
Week 12	Walk 5 minutes, jog 14 minutes, walk 4 minutes. Repeat 2 times.
Week 13	Walk 5 minutes, jog 15 minutes, walk 2 minutes. Repeat 2 times.
Week 14	Walk 5 minutes. Jog 30 minutes.

Thermoregulate, in other words, Sweat!

Some people think that sweating is gross or that it is uncomfortable to sweat. Actually, it makes me feel good to work up a healthy sweat. Sweating is the body's way to cool itself naturally. Sweating is healthy, natural and nothing to be concerned about. On the other hand, a trainer will become very alarmed if someone is exercising intensely and not sweating. Just like a car engine, if the working engine (your body) does not cool itself down, it will burn up!

At rest, our average body temperature is 98.6. Some people may actually be a degree lower. When you begin to exercise, your body temperature may rise as much as 3 degrees or to almost 102 degrees Fahrenhiet!

As your body temperature begins to rise, small blood vessels in the skin expand and draw heated blood to the skin surface as the body's water begins to escape through the pores. As the circulating air evaporates the sweat, it pulls heat away from the superficial blood vessels. The cooled blood then recirculates back down through skin layers into the body and begins to cool the core. Sweat is not just the water you drank coming through your pores to cool your core temperature down, but a nice mix of water, urea, uric acid, amino acids, ammonia, sugar, lactic acid, and ascorbic acid. I will discuss the benefits of sweating in detail more in the chapter on Alternative Approaches.

Dehydration occurs long before we are thirsty. For the asthmatic, water consumption is especially important so the lungs and the heart can work efficiently and without strain. The body's energy systems work in a fluid environment; your muscles, heart, lungs and blood all need water to keep them in chemical balance. If too much water is lost and drawn away from the muscles, blood volume decreases, which means the heart has to labor much harder to supply the same energy level.

A note on children and thermoregulation. Childrens' abilities to cool their bodies through sweating are different from those of teenagers and adults. Children have a higher threshold for triggering sweating and produce less sweat through their sweat glands. Therefore, they will not react and have the same symptoms as an exercising adult. I never deny a child a drink of water when I train them. I watch their complexion and their eyes to see if there is any change. In addition, if the child has been sick with a cold or has recently been having bouts with asthma and is just returning to exercise, I will always make the child drink a little more. I always keep 3 ounce cups on the water cooler so they do not over indulge, either. Make sure that whoever is working with your child understands these differences.

Breathing Squats

If you do no other exercise in this chapter, do this one. This exercise is probably one of the oldest strength-and-testosterone building exercises in the world of physical fitness. Long before the advent of anabolic steroids and strength-and size-building supplements such as creatine, there were breathing squats. Very few people

Air Passages: Exercise

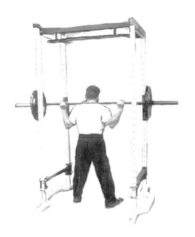

still know what breathing squats are. Most people my age and older who follow the "iron game" (a term used by devotees to weight training) have heard of them, and even in that population, very few actually practice them with any regularity. You will not find people doing breathing squats at Bally's or Scandinavian, as they are not pretty. They are painful, they will make you hurt, and they work like nothing else ever invented, for a price.

Why would you want to torture yourself with an exercise like this? Well the body, like it or not, works on a very simple premise. If you want it to get stronger, faster, more efficient, more flexible, or if you just plain want to change the look of your body, you have to challenge it to do so. It will only give you the results you want through time invested and consistency of action. You must push it ever so slightly out of your comfort zone or it will always remain complacent, or worse, never change.

Weighted breathing squats are extremely demanding on your lungs, your heart, and your body. Therefore don't do them as your first exercise with a heavy weight on your back. This may induce a sudden change in tidal volume of the lungs which will spin you into an exercise induced asthma attack faster than anything I know. It's time for the weighted bar breathing squats only after a good sweat is rolling off you.

If you are a severe asthmatic, it's best to do a simple test run of breathing squats while holding a large phonebook for 25 - 40 repetitions instead of the weighted bar. When you can do this test without breathlessness, progress to the weighted breathing squats.

You will need some special equipment for weighted breathing squats. A squat rack or power rack, an Olympic bar and plates, and a spotter. You also must have a realistic idea of how much weight you can lift with a back squat (the barbell resting on the back of your shoulders) for one time or one repetition. Once you know the maximum amount of weight in pounds you can lift one time, use a percentage of that weight to perform your desired number of repetitions. The recommended percentage is 85% of a one-repetition maximum. The weight with which you can drop down into a full squat position with (buttocks parallel with the knees) and then come back up to an erect posture, is called 1 repetition maximum. We will take .85 times that weight to figure how much weight to put on the bar.

For example, let's say you can do a back squat with 200 pounds of weight (including the bar) for one repetition. We would calculate: 200 lbs. x .85 = 175 lbs. for 85% of a one repetition maximum.

The exercise itself is relatively simple. Begin by standing in a squat rack with the bar loaded to 85% of your 1 repetition maximum. Always have the safety pins placed right below a full parallel squat position so that if anything were to happen they will catch the weight and it won't break your legs or worse. Next shoulder the bar so that it sits low on your back, across the trapezes muscle, with your hands spread wide on the bar itself. Take a deep breath and drop down to parallel position with the weighted bar. Breath out through pursed lips as you explode upward toward an upright position. After your knees have locked out, breath in deeply (belly breathing), and exhale slowly through pursed lips 3 times. Perform the next repetitions by inhaling deep, squatting down to parallel (knees parallel to the buttocks), exhaling as you push up to standing position. Remember to keep your head up as you squat down. This will keep your spine in correct postural alignment. Perform this exercise for 25 repetitions in this fashion. By the end of 15 repetitions you should be breathing pretty hard and your heart should feel like you are doing an aerobic workout. Your legs should also feel tired and you may wonder if you are going to get the last 10 repetitions.

Want to know a little trick to get through the tough exercises? Start to count backwards; this way you don't get so wrapped up in how many more you have to do, but in how few you have left. If you do not have a squat rack at your gym or home, hold on to a pair of dumbbells and do the breathing squats.

What else to do if you don't have a squat rack..........

Barbell Pullovers

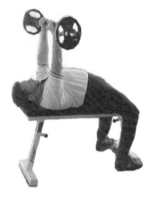

You can do this exercise with a chambered exercise bar sometimes called a curved exercise bar. This bar takes the pressure off the wrists. This is an old-time exercise to promote the stretching of the fascia located around the intercostals. If you remember, the intercostals are the muscles located near the rib cage and are used primarily by the chest breathers. It is important to develop these muscles; they need to be strong in the advent of an asthma attack. This exercise can also help to expand your ribcage, which will reduce how sore your ribs can get after a prolonged asthma attack.

You will need a flat exercise bench for this exercise. I must warn you, this exercise has a way of sneaking up on you. You will be performing the exercise easily for 8 or 9 reps and wondering if you are using enough weight, and all at once the muscles will start to fatigue and you will wonder if you can complete the set.

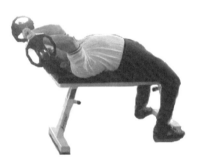

It is best if someone can hand the bar to you while you are lying on the bench. Take the bar with a narrow grip and press it out to arms length above your chest. Now begin to lower the bar back toward your forehead and past the back of your head, down as far as you can stretch it comfortably. Keep the arms bent, elbows pointed toward your feet, and inhale as deeply as you can on the descending portion of the exercise.

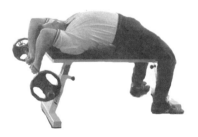

As you begin to exhale slowly through pursed lips, bring the bar back over your forehead, over your chest and stop about nipple level. Do not lock your arms out above your chest. This exercise will also work the triceps muscle (the back of your arm) extremely well. Do about 15 to 25 repetitions of this exercise after your breathing squats for an enhanced burn.

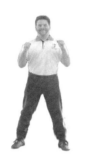 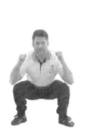 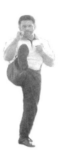

SQUAT KICK

Get ready!

Full Squat

Kick

Squat Kicks

This exercise is a martial arts warmup move that I absolutely love.

Begin by standing with your feet a little wider than shoulder width and pointing straight ahead. As in the breathing squats, keep your head up, and drop down into a parallel squat position. While coming back up to the standing position begin to bring your knee to your chest, and then extend your foot out straight in front of you. This is like the front snap kick or front kick in the martial arts. Squat down again to parallel, come up the same way, only this time alternate your kicking leg. You keep squatting and alternating kicking legs until you have reached 30 repetitions (15 per leg). Try not hurry this move; you really want to stretch the legs by doing a complete squat and by extending the kicking leg as far out as you can by pushing your hip out each time you kick.

Stomach and Abdominal Work

The stomach is the key to correct asthmatic breathing and the cornerstone of all strength and conditioning of the body. In fact, it is the cornerstone of health in general. Every athlete I know works his or her stomach muscles. Golfers, gymnasts, martial artists, and rock climbers all do extensive abdominal work. In Asia, the stomach is the focal point of the person, while the west locates it in the heart. We have sayings such as ""home is where the heart is" and "a broken heart." The irony is that in Asia, the stomachs are flat and there is no heart disease, at least prior to the Americanization of China with Big Macs and fast food.

Most people would like to have a flat stomach and a six-pack of muscle around their midsection, but very few of us do. What we can accomplish, however, is strong stomach muscles and, as a by-product, have a strong center of gravity. What does that mean? No lower back pain!

Creating a Super Strong Back that will Never Break

If one word causes empathy from the majority of us, it is "backache." Truth is, most of us have had a "back episode." In fact, almost 80 % of the population will have back trouble some time in their adult life. Out of ten people who have chronic medical conditions defined as limiting their activities, four of those are back victims. Backache is number two only to headaches as the most common medical complaint, and only the common cold causes more people to miss work! [2]

As a former personal trainer, I hear many of my clients tell me of their back pains when taking their medical histories. Here is some insight on back pain gathered from my research and my experience.

First, some risk factors to consider:

Genetics: if your mother or father have been diagnosed with intervertebral disc disease, or slipped vertebrae or herniated disks, chances are you might have it too, because these connections seem to run in families.

Job: If you spend at least half of your working hours driving a car or SUV, you are three times as likely as the average worker to end up with a herniated disk. This percentage increases dramatically if you are operating heavy equipment (backhoes, bulldozers, etc…) or driving trucks over 1 ton. It is the constant vibration that does this damage to the spine. If you sit and drive for prolonged periods, this is an accident waiting to happen! Also at risk are individuals who sit for prolonged periods, such as data entry or computer professionals.

It is interesting to note here that in cultures where people take up squatting positions frequently throughout the day, there appears to be less back pain.

In addition, people who have lower back pain are typically very tight. I mean that they lack flexibility in almost every direction. In contrast, watch a couple of 4 or 5 year olds play for a few minutes. Notice as they sit directly back on their knees, fold themselves in half with no spinal discomfort, do backbends and somersaults; their ability to roll and bend is truly amazing. Unfortunately, I start to see muscle, tendon and fascia tightness as early as age 10! By the time we reached age 40, we have had plenty of time to acquire injuries, limit our exercise and stretching, gain extra weight around our middle, and constrict our muscles in a multitude of ways.

In the martial arts classes that I teach, we spend a great deal of time stretching. We stretch only after a thorough warmup that gets everyone sweating, even in the dead of winter. Stretching performed without warming the tissues of the body can result in further injury and complicate matters significantly.

Paramount as well for a healthy back is the tone and strength of the torso. The waist/lumbar area does not contain any structural support in the form of bone mass, except for the spinal column. The only means of support is the musculature of the abdominal area and many the diverse muscle groups and layers of back muscle. These muscle groups are key for holding the back structurally in alignment. If this area becomes deconditioned and loses muscle tone, the entire spinal column becomes at risk for injury (back pain, herniated disks etc.). Using structured exercise and stretching programs, I have seen many of my clients improve their quality of life and alleviate back pain completely.

Back care and prevention are the first components of a good exercise program and should be included in everyone's daily activities. Start your son or daughter doing this before they are a teenager to give them a good solid muscle foundation. They will thank you later. It takes but a few minutes a day to do the preventative maintenance, which can go a long way in preventing back injury and pain.

Jack Knives

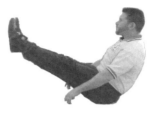

This is the king of all stomach exercises, as it really works the upper and the lower abs. Begin by relaxing your neck muscles. Remember we are exercising our abs, not our necks and shoulders here. Keep a space at all times between the chin and your chest (think about holding an apple between your chin and chest). This will allow proper air space so that you can breath normally while doing the exercise. As you come up, think about lifting your shoulders and not your head. Lift your feet at the same time and come up to form a "V" shape. Hold it there for a moment and then slowly lower back down to the starting position.

For an advanced option, or if you have a strong stomach, do not allow your feet to touch. As you lower your body down again, keep the feet together and 4 inches off the ground. Try to work up to 25 repetitions in a row, or as many as you can do.

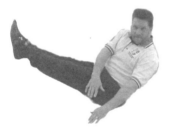

Side to Side Jack Knives

This exercise is almost the same as the regular jackknives except for one important difference. All the rules for regular jackknives apply here (head, chin, etc) but you must rotate the body on the up position to one side or the other. It is best to alternate sides with each repetition, otherwise you might develop cramping.

Dips

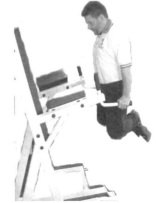

Dips are among the exercise staples of many a bodybuilder, strength athlete or anyone truly interested in physical fitness. This exercise is best performed on dipping bars, but you can improvise by using two very strong chair backs placed with the seats in opposite directions. The key to doing this exercise, and all exercises for that matter, is to do a full range of motion. In other words, allow your body to go as deeply as it possibly can and to straighten out fully at the top of the motion. Make sure you do this movement without snapping the joints at the top or bouncing at the bottom, otherwise you will eventually injure the joint capsule. This movement allows your body to stretch the muscles, tendons and ligaments in a full range while exercising. A muscle trained in full range of motion will always be stronger and less prone to injury.

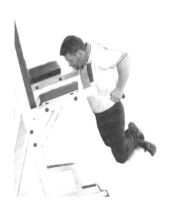

A stretched muscle is a stronger muscle and faster muscle, especially in the martial arts or combative sports.

Pushups!!!

I love pushups! No, I don't hold any world record, but I do like the way they make me feel. I have discovered or invented, I am not sure which, a number of ways to do pushups. Many of these variations came from martial arts training.

I think we all know how to do pushups, but here are a few pointers that can make them more fun to do. First, make sure that you do a full range of motion. In my martial arts classes, I have women, men and children. About 3% do pushups correctly all the time without being reminded. They are very difficult to do right, and if you do them right, you won't be able to do as many as your friends do. This of course is if you are interested in numbers more than results. Second, for a real pump or burn of the muscles, contract the pectorals (chest muscles) at the top of the movement. This will give you a full feeling in your chest as you push more blood into the area. Third, make sure that your hands are placed so that your thumbnails are aligned where the pectorals and the armpit meet. This will give a slight stretch to the muscle and ensure full contraction of the muscle. Fourth, make sure you touch your chest to the ground each time gently. No bouncing off the ground here! Fifth, keep the legs straight, knees locked and the ankles touching. Do not allow your thighs to touch the ground. Sixth, contract your abdominals to keep your midsection from collapsing or sagging downward. Squeeze your stomach like someone was about to punch you in the stomach, and keep it tight throughout the entire movement. Last but not least, keep your gluteous maximus (butt) down and parallel with the rest of your body.

Regular Breathing Pushups

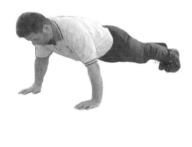

If you are not strong enough to do military pushups yet (on your toes with legs off the ground) then try to do pushups with your knees down, toes touching the ground. A rule of thumb here: the farther your legs are from your hands; the more difficult the push-up becomes. The closer the hands are to the knees the easier it becomes. The difference between my pushups and regular military pushups is that I use specialized breathing techniques while doing the exercise.

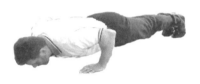

Starting from the up position (see photo) you will begin to inhale deeply into the abdomen as you descend in the lowered position. Hold for 1 second and then begin to exhale as you ascend toward your starting position. This is one complete push-up. You will notice that these are done much more methodically than other types of fast-paced frenzied pushups you see in exercise tapes or classes. The concept is to breath in deeply while expanding the pectoral (chest) / ribcage area. This will be true with all the push-up variations that follow.

Wide Breathing Pushups

WARNING: If you have rotator cuff problems or other shoulder problems, please do not attempt these.

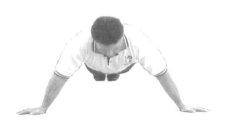

These are the same as regular breathing pushups, only place your hands about a foot farther apart than for regular pushups. Turn the hand so that they abduct or turn outward away from the body which will stimulate the side portion of your chest. This is noticeably different than the previous push-up.

Close Breathing Pushups

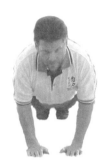

WARNING: This exercise is hard on the wrists and forearms, so if you have problems in this area, please take heed.

Again, the same rules apply here as for regular pushups, but bring the hands in alignment under your nipples.

One note on all the pushups: for an additional stretch and expansion in the chest and shoulder area, you can place both of your hands on thick phonebooks to assist in a deeper stretch. This opens the muscle groups around the chest/shoulder/ribs that control breathing.

Fist Breathing Pushups

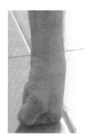

This is a martial arts form of pushups, traditionally performed to strengthen the wrist for punching. Make sure the fist is tight and you bend the wrist slightly so that the first two knuckles, (the index finger and the middle finger) are taking the pressure. These two bones of the hand are sturdier than the other finger/knuckles in the hand.

Finger Pushups

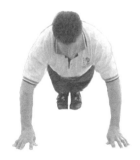

This is a tough one. Assume regular push-up position with your knees down, form your hands into a claw (like you are gripping a ball about 6 inches in diameter) and try to keep this position while you touch your chest to the ground. This builds enormous strength in the fingers and hands.

Triangle Breathing Pushups

This movement is for the triceps muscle (the back of your arm), which actually comprises 2/3 of the girth of your arm. The triceps is active when you push or punch. Move the hands into a triangle position, making sure the two index fingers touch and the thumbs touch. Extend the arms out to a 45-degree angle. You may have to start on your knees for this one.

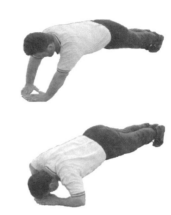

Decline Breathing Pushups

WARNING: If you have high blood pressure, DO NOT do this version. This pushes a lot of blood into the head region and causes a lot of pressure.

This push-up is done by placing your feet on a sturdy chair or bench. This will lift the feet well above the head and place additional pressure on the shoulders, chest and triceps. This particular push-up is good for defining the lower part of the pectoral muscle.

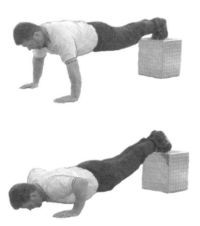

Chinese Breathing Pushups

This is a unique kind of push-up and a stretching movement for the legs and groin. Do this on a non-slip surface so you can control how far your legs spread.

Stand about shoulder width apart and slowly move your feet out to the sides. Move downward until your feet are as far as they can go comfortably. At this point the push-up starts. Place your palms down in front of you in line with your shoulders. Rock forward, bringing your chest to the ground; arch your back as you come up and rock back to your beginning position. Your legs should not move, and you will feel a stretch on the inside of the thighs and groin.

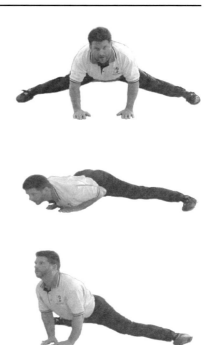

Stretching

One of the least talked about and misunderstood fitness topics is stretching. The stretching I talk about here is full body movement, constant motion through a full range of motion. In fact, it is its own little exercise routine unto itself.

Whereas the previously exercises were quite demanding, this group of exercises is very beneficial for the frail, the newcomer to exercise, and the asthmatic.

Let us begin with some basics first. Forget about the "no pain no gain" theory. That concept definitely does not apply here. Avoid all feeling of pain when stretching. A pulling feeling may be felt when stretching tight muscles, but it should never be unbearable.

One other point about stretching that fails to be mentioned. Relax the muscles that you are trying to stretch. This concept sounds like common sense, but is rarely achieved in practice. In my many years of training clients, I have seen many people stretching and holding a posture through shear muscle contraction, rather than through relaxing and allowing their body to elongate.

There is a plethora of stretching routines and techniques out there that can make stretching more complicated than it is. However,

Air Passages: Exercise

simple is always better in most of life's adventures. Move the body slowly and with purpose in many different directions without pain. How is that for a simple prescription?

Notice that you may be tighter on one side of your body than the other. This is normal. Moreover, I have found that the dominant side of the body is usually stronger, but has a more limited range of motion. The non-dominant side is weaker usually, but more flexible.

Before you stretch, make sure you are warm and sweating or thoroughly warmed up. Do this stretching routine after your squats and pushups and/or after your treadmill routine. If you are not properly warmed-up and have your body temperature elevated before you stretch, you can actually cause damage to the very muscle fibers you are trying to elongate. By definition, "warmed up" means that the capillaries in the areas to be stretched have dilated and blood has moved into the area. The blood bathes and cushions the area against microscopic muscle tears that eventually can lead to the loss of range of motion or stiffness. The following stretches are adapted from my martial arts training and can also be done in sequence for a complete stand alone workout. Again, please remember the importance of a good warmup for asthmatics.

Backstroke Stretch

WARNING: This may be difficult for those with tight shoulders.

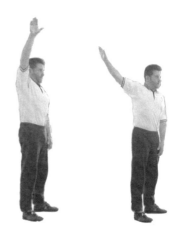

Begin by raising your arm over your head, thumb pointed upward. As the hand reaches straight over your head, rotate the hand so that the thumb will be pointing in front of you, turning the thumb back towards the front of your body. Keep the arm as straight as possible and try not to let it vary from perpendicular position. Repeat with the other arm.

Slap Sides

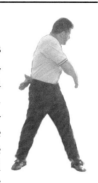

This a martial arts warmup exercise that starts to loosen the waist, slightly stretch the intercostals, and loosen the shoulders or deltoids. Begin with your feet shoulder width apart, knees slightly bent. Relax the waist, arms at the sides for now, and begin to move the waist (not the legs) as if you were about to look behind you to the left and then to the right. As you start to feel more and more stretched and loose, increase the speed of turning until your arms start to take flight by the sheer momentum of your movement. The hands will begin to "slap" the sides of waist if you allow your arms to become loose as well.

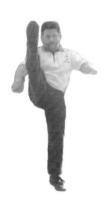

Front Stretch Kick

This movement is similar to a place kick in football. You may want to hold on to something until you can trust your balance. Step back with your right leg and allow your left leg to bend at the knee. Gently swing the right leg up as high as you can, while keeping the leg locked at the knee joint and pulling the toes back toward the shin bone. This will stretch the muscles of the hamstring (back of thigh) and the calf muscles (gastrocnemius and soleus).

The Cat

Step 1: Table position: Kneel down on all fours with your legs shoulder width apart, your arms spaced in line with your knees and hands on the floor directly below your shoulders, and your head in line with your spine. Your back is flat, like a table.

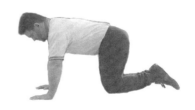

Step 2: Inhale deeply, using your diaphragm; open your chest and expand it as you sink your back and your stomach towards the floor. Raise your head up as your sitting bones tip towards the ceiling. Breathe deeply while allowing the front of the body to stretch open. Hold the breath momentarily.

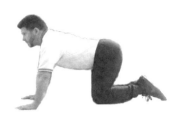

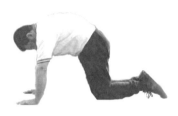

Step 3: Breathe out evenly, pulling your stomach in towards your spine. Slowly arch your back as high as you can while dropping your head between your arms. Your sitting bones will roll down and point towards the ground. You are like an angry cat, arching its back. Hold this position for a few moments, letting the muscle around the ribs contract, and pull the abdominal muscles in.

Wag the Dog's Tail

Still kneeling in the Table position, you are going to arch your spine from side to side, like a comma or letter C. Look over your right shoulder, towards your feet, keeping the back flat but curving to the side. Your hips will move to the left. Your feet may move to the right. Inhale. Slowly, repeat the other side, and exhale.

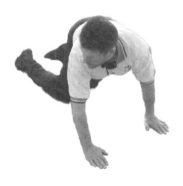

Thread the Needle

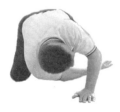

This exercise really stretches my neck and shoulders and intercostals all in one movement. While in Table position, raise the right arm up to the ceiling, while twisting, opening and exposing the chest to that side. Inhale. Then take your right arm and thread it between your left arm and left leg. As you pull your arm through, like threading a needle, come to rest on your right shoulder. Exhale. This is now stretching the torso, neck and shoulder. Now, the left hand then comes up to the ceiling and opens the chest. Inhale, hold, then exhale. Slowly, bring your left arm down to the floor, and return to Table position. Repeat on the other side. Breathe deeply, but normally and allow your body to relax and lengthen.

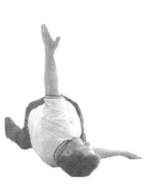

Downward Facing Dog

Start from Table position. Curl your toes under, "point" your sitting bones toward the ceiling, breathe in and slide and push your feet backward. Exhale, push your sitting bones towards the ceiling, lift your knees off the floor, straighten your legs, heels coming towards the floor. Press into the floor with the heel of your hands, like a push-up. Press your index fingers and thumbs into the floor, taking the weight away from the pinkie edge of your hands. As your hands press into the floor, lengthen your arms away from your wrists. Rotate your pelvis forward to lift your sitting bones away from your heels. Lift your hips high into the air, stretching them away from your waist and toward the wall behind you. Press your heels downward while lifting the arches of your feet. Relax your head and neck muscles. When ready, return to Table position.

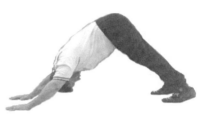

Modified Fish

This movement really stretches the rib cage and opens the throat. This is a good stretch for the brachial plexus, a muscle commonly tight in asthmatics, and just feels good as it counters our normal posture as well as the downward facing dog position. Begin by lying on the floor on your back, legs straight and arms by your sides, hands palm down. Next, inhale and lift your trunk slowly while moving your arms back, bending the elbows so the weight supports your shoulders. Hollow out your scapula area while letting your head fall back.

Holding the breath momentarily, move your elbows slowly outward until the soft spot of your head rests on the floor. Remember to keep your buttocks down and breath slowly with the belly for about 30 seconds. Slowly return to lying flat on the floor, and feel what muscles have been gently stretched by this movement.

Pierce the Sky

Note: if you have lumbar, disk, or lower back problems Do NOT try this.

Stand erect, feet shoulder width apart. Expel the breath, and then inhaling slowly, swing both arms up in the air over your head while pushing your hips forward. Place your hands together as if in prayer, breathe normally and allow the stretch to happen. Then drop the your hands behind your back, while simultaneously opening the chest and shoulders to the sky above you. Feel the stretch in the abdominals, ribs and chest. Breathe through the nose normally for several breaths.

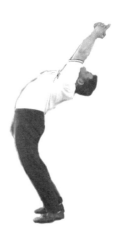

Half Moon

This is basically a side-to-side stretch done with your palms pressed together overhead with your arms fully extended. Inhale in the center, and as you exhale, bend to the side and feel the muscles stretch along the rib cage, back and hips.

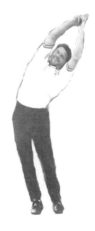

Plies

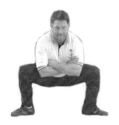

This is similar to the squat position, except your foot position will change. You may want to hold onto something to stabilize yourself until you get used to this way of moving. Stand a little wider than shoulder width apart and point your toes out to right angles of their normal position. Now squat down slowly and feel the muscles in the inner thigh begin to stretch and work. This is a wonderful exercise and stretch that is similar to ballet movements, and you know what great legs ballet dancers have.

Trembling Horse

Of all the movements listed, this is probably the simplest, but the hardest to perform. I say this because this stretch works your inner fascia and requires total relaxation of your body from head to toe. It actually works through a vibration that you send through your body. The effect is similar to an electrostimulation machine used in physical therapy, only it is self-administered.

Begin by relaxing your hands, then wrists, then elbows, and then shoulders. This being accomplished, and that is a big accomplishment, start to slightly oscillate your entire arm from fingertips to shoulders, within a very small circumference. The next step is to start this small oscillation at your hips and extend upward to your torso and ending with your head. Finally, put the two movements together and do them simultaneously. Take your time and truly relax, and you will begin to feel your body release from the inside out.

Martial Arts Training

> *"You will never do anything in this world without courage, it is the greatest quality of the mind next to honor"*
>
> *James Allen*

The martial arts are an enormously important part of my life that I believe can benefit any child or adult who is compromised in any physical or emotional way. I have such faith in the martial arts that

I highly recommend that everyone try it for a couple months. If you don't like the training or the teacher, please try another style of martial art or change teachers. As the styles vary, so too do the organization of classes and the ratio of physical to mental training, so make an effort to find the right fit.

The Brief History of Inner Strength Martial Arts

My personal journey in the martial arts has heavily influenced my views on exercise, longevity, mental and even spiritual development. I began my Judo training back in 1965, when there were very few, if any, children taking the martial arts. Many people have seen Judo in the Olympics, so I won't go into detail about its training methods. The teachers at that time were mostly military personal who learned their art overseas during the war. The schools were a lot different then. Discipline was strict and unforgiving. Even though I was a child, I was expected to keep up as best as I could. After all, this was a man's arena...no place for children, weak men, or women. There were no women training in our class at that time. Classes consisted of 1/2 hour of calisthenics, then tumbling and break-fall drills were done. Next came the worst part of training, when the seniors threw you over and over again, so they could practice their judo throws. Of course, you were supposed to practice your break-falls at this time. Next we sparred and sparred and sparred some more. After class was finished, we were expected to clean the dojo and the toilets, black belts and white belts (newcomers) worked side by side doing this. It was a very humbling experience. It required team effort and camaraderie. We also had to press our own uniforms and make sure they were clean. (To be honest my mother did that part for me). Whew! I did this kind of training for quite a while, but many times my asthma got so bad I couldn't train. My instructor had seen something in me, however, and realized that martial arts was everything to me. He did something very unusual at that time and trained me privately. Sometimes only 15 or 20 minutes was all I could tolerate on days when my asthma was exacerbated, but that was enough. I loved martial arts and I loved the Zazen meditation that was taught to me because it made me feel special. I felt special because the other judukas were not getting the privilege of private Zazen training with the master (in the martial arts world this is a privilege and honor). Moreover, this was something I could do that they were not versed in! It was a gift from my instructor, who realized I needed meditation more than I needed to practice throws and break-falls. It's all I wanted to do in life! I received my black belt unofficially when I was 14. Unofficially because children weren't allowed to have a true black belt because they were not yet physically and mentally mature.

Judo eventually lost its appeal for me (but not Zazen meditation). I wanted something that worked with Qi or life force energy more deeply in order to build on my foundation of meditation. I instinctively knew that my own progress toward health and longevity required that I study and practice Qi cultivation through meditation. So I began my long journey searching for the "ideal instructor." I tried local instructors but they didn't offer what I wanted. I continued to train myself through high school graduation and into college. In college I met a number of people who had trained in many different styles of fighting as well as different instructors. We exchanged ideas and trained together informally, and in this way I added styles to my own repertoire. Some of the styles were from Kempo, Tae kwon do and Gung fu.

I finally met a Tang Soo Do instructor who spoke broken English (he had just come over from Korea) who seemed to posses knowledge of Qi and hard QiGong techniques. He used to demonstrate his powers by sticking motorcycle spokes through his arms, attaching buckets of sand to the spokes, and then lifting the buckets holding his arms out straight and parallel to the ground. As the buckets of sand left the ground, his flesh never tore! Not only did his pain control impress me, but he did not bleed after pulling the spokes back out! This was just the sort of control I wanted over my body and mind. I signed up for lessons, but they reminded me of the old strict training again. I remember one class where I was being taught by one of the higher belts. He told me once to keep my hands up. Concentrating on the new technique he was teaching me, I let my hands drop only for a moment. The next thing I knew I was on my back with a burning pain in my chest and I couldn't breath. He had hit me full force in the solar plexus. I can remember him saying " I just saved your life, in the street you would be dead. I will only tell you one time to do something basic, and you better do it".

I knew that the discipline here was what I wanted. I received my black belt from Huang Kee, the founder of Tang Soo Do, in 1984 after a rigorous 2 day test. I continued with this same instructor for a total of 14 years and ran schools for him in addition to my "full time" job. He desperately wanted me to quit my job and open several schools of my own, but I didn't see a lot of income potential with his system. Eventually his format of teaching changed to a "safer" way of training, but still he did not divulge any of his secret Qi techniques to me or anyone else. Soon I was looking for another instructor, and I began to understand what Bruce Lee had always said, "absorb only what is useful, disregard the rest."

It was about this time that I started training in Chen Taijiquan. Chen style is slow moving series of movements designed to be slightly more martial than other forms of taijiquan, but it was a nice transition into the internal martial arts for me. This internal art was beautiful to watch and fun to do, but my instructor did not know the fighting application for the form. I enjoyed the training and the feel of Qi flowing through my body because it felt so different from the hard styles that I was used to. I desperately wanted to learn the internal fighting arts and the power of Qi cultivation but there was no instructor in my area who trained in Baguazhang or Hsing Yi.

I drove to North Carolina for a life-changing seminar on a fighting style called Silat, a very vicious form of jungle warfare. There I met Victor Dethoras, Bob Venetta, and Sam. Victor was from Colorado, and so was Bob. Sam was from Pennsylvania, my home state. I was introduced to Tonkat and had a brief exposure to the advanced style of Silat. Tonkat had everything: low kicks, vicious elbows, headbutts and knees, and a very unique system of takedowns and groundfighting I had never seen before. I was in love. I continued to drive every weekend to West Virginia to train with Sam. Sam was already a black belt in Silat and was learning Tonkat from Victor. Sam and I ran seminars every 3 to 6 months bringing in either Victor, or Bob to teach a seminar. We paid for their airfare by charging fees for a weekend seminar of 8 hours. Bob usually stayed at Sam's house, and after the seminar, we would pick his brain until the wee hours of the morning, and then get up and train again at the seminar. Sam and I would have enough new information to go over until we could fly them back again. Sam got married and had a child and well, things obviously had to change. No more seminars, no more training with Sam every weekend, and again I was forced to find another instructor. I needed more information and I didn't feel "complete" yet.

I was in my late twenties now, had a good job in computer programming, and had vacation time coming. I heard about "death camps" being held on a several hundred acre farm somewhere in the Smokey Mountains. Here, martial artists from all over the world trained for 2 weeks, 12 hours a day, in every aspect of combat. Knife fighting, stick fighting, and various firearms were also taught. Many of the people attending this camp were professional bodyguards, bounty hunters, and people who depended on their martial arts skill to survive in life-and-death situations. These camps were by invitation only, and I had a contact to get in. Guess where I went on vacation? Not to Disney! I signed up, and it changed my thinking about martial arts and self-defense forever. I won't go into a lot of detail about the camps, but it was here that I truly learned what worked in reality. The camps were brutal, exhausting, and fun, but no place for the feint of heart. At the camp, were people trained in so many styles of martial arts, some very exotic, some, of which I had never heard of, and they all traded ideas and concepts. The camaraderie was very high, and egos were put on a shelf for two weeks. People here were training to absorb and learn new skills, nothing more. There truly was something for every interest and expertise. It was there that I met Tim Tacket. He was one of the few men who had personally trained with Bruce Lee, and before that was the first white man to achieve a black sash in Hsing-I Gung fu. Hsing-I is one of only three internal (using Qi power instead of brute force) martial arts from China. Internal martial arts not only teach physical fighting concepts, but also about energy systems in the body that can be used for healing. In China, the local martial arts master, armed with this knowledge, is considered the local primary care physician, because he understands all that classically trained acupuncturists do, and then some. Although I met Tim only a few times, he had a profound impact on my future thinking. I continued to train at these camps for several years until the farm was sold and the camp disbanded.

When I was thirty, I realized that the weak link in my ability was grappling. I had heard about the Gracie family and their offer of $10,000 to anyone who could beat them in a no-holds barred fight. This intrigued me. I flew to California to start my training with the Gracies and I met Royce and Rorian Gracie. The two are brothers who carry on a system of Brazilian fighting perfected by their father Helio. My first experience with them was a very pleasurable one. I had arranged for two weeks of vacation to check out California and dedicate myself to training. I worked out a deal to take as many as four, 2-hour classes a day plus private lessons with Royce for the entire two weeks. I also joined Gold's gym, where Royce worked out. At this time, he was preparing to compete in the first Ultimate Fighting Championship. What I liked about the Gracie system is that, unlike Judo, this martial art really does rely on leverage and not brute strength. Economy of motion and skill are their claim to fame. Classes were all about fighting. Time is allowed to explore a new technique, but right after, you sparred many different students to see if you could use the new move in combat. One technique would be the focus of the entire two-hour class. Talk about perfectionists! Most of the guys training at this time were ex-wrestlers and big. I was the smallest guy at the Gracie academy, but I never let that stop me. I continued to train with the Gracies until I heard about their cousins, the Machados, who also were in California. The Machados were probably lesser known (at this time anyway) than their famous cousins, but equally as skilled. Carlos Machado, who is my teacher, is also teaching Chuck Norris, of Walker Texas Ranger fame. Carlos is a very humble man, but lethal. The Machados' school is much smaller than the Gracie's, therefore I got a lot more attention in class. For this reason only, I continued to train with Carlos. For the next several years, my vacation time was spent training with both of these families. This brings me to the present; I am now somewhat content with my knowledge of fighting (finally). In addition, I have found several teachers in internal martial arts and QiGong that I plan on dedicating the rest of my martial arts career. I will eternally have teachers, learn and ask questions because there is so much to explore and it's fun to broaden the mind.

Martial arts, along with my exercise routines, was a method of self-development that addressed my need to heal my physically weak body, develop my breath and Qi, and give me the self-confidence and focus of mind that, in my opinion, could not have been matched by any other method. I encourage any asthmatic to seek out a martial arts instructor who has character and understanding enough to help you on your individual journey. My path was a long and winding one to get where I am today. I have found in hindsight that all martial arts systems are great, but the teacher is the biggest variable to look at. A teacher who "walks the walk," that remains centered and true to himself, who is humble and caring and places honor above monetary gain is indeed truly the master.

(1)Environmental Protection Agency "130 Cities Exceed Lead Levels for Drinking Water" Environmental News (Oct 1992)
(2)Perspectives in Exercise Science and Sport Medicine, Vol 2, Youth Exercise and Sport, Carl V. Gisolfi, David R. Lamb

CHAPTER 8

Alternative Approaches

Why Alternative Approaches?

Human beings are funny creatures, I think. When we are first diagnosed with a particular ailment or serious disease, there is a part of us that denies having it. It is like a defense mechanism that says "ignore it and it will go away." This phase is a negative one, of course, and it varies in length from minutes to years depending on the patient. Some, however, may never acknowledge the disease until it becomes too late to treat it effectively. Parents, best friends, even physicians and pharmacists can recommend treatments, or even write prescriptions for treatments, but until the person is committed to helping himself, none of these things work. Treatment can fail because the treatment plan is wrong, but it can also fail because the patient didn't put in the effort necessary or even because the patient lacked a mindful or positive intent. The Chinese call this part of the mind the "Yi" and I have come to believe in its ability to change a person's future. I will discuss this in much more detail later. I believe there are three positive phases of treatment one goes through when one is willing to listen, learn and fight an ailment.

Phase One: Traditional. One seeks out a traditional allopathic medical doctor and starts to take the medical advice seriously. If the medication states, "take every 6 hours," you begin taking the pills every 6 hours. Many times with serious illness, the treatments do not work as prescribed and need to be adjusted or changed altogether. Sometimes you need to search out another physician or specialist. You then become coordinator and coach of "the team" of physicians you are paying for. One physician may be a dermatologist and another an allergist. The physicians need to talk to each other, brainstorm and flowchart a course of action. The first phase includes the willingness to patiently go along with all the changes and recommendations "the team" may suggest. On occasion, I hear of individuals who write off allopathic medicine from the beginning. I don't consider this a smart move because each discipline has something to offer. All treatments, from Tibetan medicine, to practices of Chi Kung (or QiGong), to laser surgery have their place. Sometimes it is more the practitioner than the practice that makes the difference, as I have found out. Don't be afraid to get a second opinion.

Phase Two: Alternative. Once you determine for yourself that you are responsible for your own health and well-being, your thought process and actions will change dramatically. Many times, despite the effectiveness of today's modern technology, pharmaceuticals and surgical techniques, results are not produced, or the side effects of treatment are not to the patient's liking. This becomes the second leg of the journey. This journey now has a name: we call it alternative or complementary or integrative medicine in the west. In the '60s, when I first became interested in "alternative medicine" it wasn't called that at all. In fact, it really did not have a standardized name. The people who practiced it were looked upon as hippies, freaks, belonging to some cult or religion, or "just out there." I have to admit, some of the people I consulted in the 60's and 70's were somewhat strange. I found them all very nice people, very kind, and knowledgable in their areas. Environmental consciousness seemed to be a common theme. These were the naturopaths, herbalists, and Taoist priests who had a background in Chinese medicine.

Phase Three: Personal. This phase is when you have been dealing with an ailment for quite a long period. You know the minute details and facts of the ailment through education from your physician, through self-education via reading, seminars, support groups etc., and through intuition of what works and what will not. For most people in phase three, it is a combination of the Traditional and the Alternative phases that make the best sense for them. This phase affects most patients with such chronic disease as asthma, chronic pain and life-threatening diseases like cancer.

Some people might ask "how can you ask people to rely on matters so vital as one's health on information and treatments that have not been scientifically proven"? Is all of this new-age, mind-body medicine and alternative medicine just a nostrum as a get rich scheme?

First of all, scientific standards or known 'facts' change every few years, at best. What is accepted as "fact" and science one year, may be totally disproven the following year. One hundred years ago, physicians considered that washing their hands between surgical patients was considered "unnecessary". This belief wasn't the scientific fact of its day. Advances, breakthroughs and new studies are happening daily. Some alternative therapy exists because while it may be 'scientifically unproven', it has worked for people for centuries. Perhaps empirical evidence gathered over hundreds of years is true science?

According to Time Magazine (October 1999), we originally thought there were 80,000 genes in the human body. Genes, of course, are the functional units of heredity that make each one of us look, act or feel like our fore-bearers. Now scientists have uncovered that we may have as many as 140,000 genes in the body, and only a meager 12% of DNA has been decoded so far! It is difficult for science to even imagine how complex we are, let alone analyze and decode that complexity. The more we uncover and learn about the human body, brain and mind, the less we realize that we know. All of this biology does not even touch the issue of spirituality and the role it plays in the cocktail of intertwined uniqueness we call being human.

Every one of us is unique. The following programs have had value to me. I encourage you to think about them, try them if they seem appropriate, and become inspired to seek out other forms of therapy that seem appropriate and effective for you.

Sweat Therapy

Many cultures believe that sweating is a therapy or purification of the body. Many naturopathic doctors, spas and indigenous cultures around the world have used this form of therapy for generations. The American Indians used sweat lodges and burned sweet grass to purify their bodies before combat and to help heal. We call this detoxification in the modern world, a concept that again is beginning to show promise.

Modern saunas, specifically steamed, always seem to exacerbate my asthma symptoms. However, I do like the effect of sweating and purifying myself while burning some fat calories or by taking hot baths for therapeutic purposes.

The popular press is full of articles extolling sweat therapy as a way to encourage health and to prevent or cure illness. I'm not sure about some of the claims, for example that it can prevent all forms of cancer. I believe it has much to offer for skin disorders and general detoxification and should definitely be a part of your survival kit. Moreover, several martial artists I know insist that this is an excellent way to clear the mind and prepare for competition (battle). I do think it is an excellent way for people with eczema and psoriasis to help their skin to maintain homeostasis or balance.

Sweat therapy and therapeutic baths have a long record of proven accomplishment behind them. There are many known benefits from sweat therapy. It clears the lymphatic system of congestion and removes certain heavy toxic metals including mercury, lead, aluminum, and arsenic. Sweat therapy also removes modern toxins such as those in automobile exhaust, chemical solvents, toner cartridges in printers and copiers, particle board used in new home construction, toxins in household cleaning supplies, and also the chemical residue in our food. [1]

Sweat therapy reduces the stress on the immune system, which allows the filtering plants of your body, namely the liver and kidneys, to cleanse themselves. This allows the nervous system to rejuvenate itself. The sweating and detoxification will increase your stamina, reduce blood pressure, lower cholesterol, and here is the big one: allow the body to have increased resistance to allergens.

The whole idea of sweating just makes common sense. We had to sweat more in the past, before air-conditioned cars, office buildings and homes. Labor-saving devices are the norm today. No longer do we have to cut wood or shovel coal to warm our houses. If you are tired and don't feel like doing the stairs - take the escalator or the elevator. Merge these two together and we have a phenomenon unnatural to the human body: lack of consistent sweating from exercise and purification. The only time we sweat is in the gym or on weekends working outside!

The skin is the largest organ on the human body. The skin is such a unique and extraordinary organ that I think most people take it for granted until something goes wrong. The skin is actually a semi-permeable membrane that works like a two-lane highway for protection and for expulsion of toxins and waste products. This skin permeability allows transdermal patches, herbal poultices, therapeutic baths and aromatherapy oils to penetrate and work systemically. The same skin allows the body, via certain poultices and herbals, to push out or purge toxins and waste products through the sudoriferous or sweat glands.

The skin protects you from bacteria and external toxins by the secretion of sebum (oil from the sebaceous glands), sweat, lipids and salts. When we take on more toxins than our body is able to handle through normal means, and the filtering plant called the liver is congested with toxins, the body tries to push them out through the skin. Alas, the very organ (the liver) that tries to cleanse and purge these toxins falls victim to the very substances that it is trying to clear. There are exceedingly copious quantities of chemicals, fertilizers, preservatives, drugs, water contamination, refined sugars, and processed fats and proteins pumped into our diets every day. Over time, the toxins can build up in the tissues and remain there for years before they produce any noticeable adverse affect on your health.

Sweat therapy is a wonderful way to purge the body of toxins, but it might also have a new benefit. Researchers in Germany have identified that sweat may automatically secrete a natural antibiotic onto our skin that may be the first line of defense in fighting bacteria and fungi. They have named this antibiotic Demcidin.

Sweat therapy as a therapeutic bath is a hot water bath, typically in the range of 100 to 104 degrees F. It may take you awhile to adjust to hot baths, but they are wonderful little luxuries that are so therapeutic. Always follow your sweat bath with a cool shower because a hot bath slows oxygen movement to the brain. A cool shower returns oxygen flow to normal.

Epsom Salts Baths

Epsom salts (magnesium sulfate) have been used as a therapy for a long time. As a boy, I can remember soaking my finger in Epsom salts when I had a splinter to bring the infection to a head. Epsom salts are wonderfully therapeutic for aches and pain associated with sore muscles and repetitive overuse injury. A hot bath with water as warm as you can stand it with about 5 pounds of Epsom salts will clear the lymphatic system and the energetic matrix of the body quite well. Soak for about 15 to 20 minutes, or for shorter periods if you are new to this kind of therapy. Some health coaches suggest as high as 15 or 16 pounds in the bath water. The more Epsom salts in the water, the more perspiration will occur as the osmotic pressure pulls the toxins from the fluid-base of the body. This kind of bath can drain you, so do not do this more than one time per week. For small children and very sensitive-skinned individuals, you may have to cut the concentration down by almost a half at first.

Hydrogen Peroxide Baths

Hydrogen peroxide is used in a multitude of therapies for the rejuvenation of the body. Even nature uses it, as, for example the healing water of Lourdes in France. Hydrogen Peroxide (H_2O_2) has an extra molecule of oxygen attached to it. When added to warm bath water, the extra molecule is released and to be absorbed by the body. A hydrogen peroxide bath is antibacterial, antiviral, and cleansing to the energetic body (see chapter 12 for further explanation on Chinese Medicine). It is also a good supportive practice during chemotherapy.

Use a good food grade source of hydrogen peroxide for your bath, which is a 35% solution. The supermarket version is only a 3% solution; because it is not as potent, you will need 2 to 4 pints (U.S.) in the bath. Use about 6 ounces of the food grade version in the bath. The food grade version is very concentrated, so be careful handling it, because it can irritate the skin quickly. Once diluted in the full tub, however, the food grade version is fine. Soak for about 20 minutes.

Oatmeal Baths

I find baths made from colloidal oatmeal (Aveeno is one brand name) to be very soothing to irritated skin, although they do feel as if they leave a slight film on my body. Soak for 20 minutes and then apply your moisturizer mixture of aloe vera and AmLactin.

Apple Cider Vinegar Baths

Apple cider vinegar made from unprocessed pure resources is the best choice here. Commercially made Apple Cider Vinegar loses many of the properties that make it effective. Unprocessed apple cider vinegar contains many trace minerals, such as potassium, phosphorus, magnesium, sodium, silicon and sulfur. These nourish the skin and return the skin to its natural pH level. Use 2 to 4 cups in your bath water or adjust it to your nose sensitivity. It is pungent. Soak for 20 minutes and apply the moisturizer of aloe vera and AmLactin.

Baking Soda Baths

I can remember clearly the day I was playing with my cousins at my grandmother's house in the fall. The air was cool and crisp and my asthma was hardly bothering me and I was actually running and playing outside. Well, in my excitement, I accidentally stepped on a yellow jackets nest nestled in the ground. The fall is the time of year when yellow jackets in Pennsylvania build their winter nests and are very aggressive and protective of their winter sanctuary. Within seconds, the yellow jackets had covered me from head to toe. They were in my hair, eyes, and ears…. everywhere! They were angry that I had destroyed their "winter home" and were going to make me pay. I ran screaming to my grandmother's porch, where everyone came rushing out to see what was wrong. My mother was grabbing handfuls of bees and just throwing them off my body. I know she was thinking that given my many allergies, I could swell up from anaphylactic shock and quickly die. I immediately began to swell from the massive number of bites that I had sustained. Luckily I swelled only where I had been bitten, not in my throat. Fortunately, I was not fatally allergic to them. I can also remember my grandmother making a paste of baking soda, water, and apple cider vinegar and just slathering my skin from head to toe with it. The mixture worked well; it dried up the bites and allowed me to control the itching from the hives.

Baking soda in the bath soothes irritated itching skin and allows the skin to detoxify. Use two to four pounds of baking soda in a bathtub, and soak for 20 minutes. Some people claim that our bodies pick up minute quantities of radiation from computer monitors, television screens, x-rays as well as CAT scans.[2] A bath with baking soda and natural sea salt will clear up and detoxify this condition. Use 1 or 2 equal pounds of baking soda and sea salt combined in a warm bath. Soak for 20 minutes and apply the moisturizer of aloe vera and AmLactin.

Coffee

This is one of my all time best proven methods for decreasing the symptoms of an asthma attack. A piping hot cup of coffee is one thing that is necessary for people having an asthma attack. Whether you take your rescue remedy (Albuterol) or not, I still recommend it. During an attack, I would always would make myself to drink coffee because it breaks up mucus secretions. People ask me if I put natural honey in it, or if I drink it black, or how it is prepared. The best recipe is exactly the way you like it. If you don't like coffee at all, no matter how it's prepared, then drink it black. Why add calories?

Later on, through research, I learned that caffeine has similar chemical structure to a drug called theophylline, which is a bronchodilator. Some pharmacological brand names of theophylline are Theo-Dur, Slo-bid, Theo-24, and Resbid, which you may recognize.

I drink 2 cups of coffee in the morning for medicinal purposes (I'm sure you heard that before) about 45 minutes apart. This gives me enough time to get 16 oz. of water into my body before my weight-training / stretching workout. If you have sinusitis or heavy mucous in the nose every time you wake up, this also is good therapy paired with the snorting of saline solution below.

Mucous

The next few sections deal with ways to release the copious amounts of mucous that we allergy/asthma people produce. The average adult produces one quart of mucous per day in their sinuses alone. If we have allergies or asthma, we produce so much more. Remember, we are efficient creatures!

Saline Wash

Snorting a mixture of saline solution and other ingredients into the nose and then blowing out the mixture along with mucous that has accumulated overnight can be a great therapy for the asthmatic and those with rhinitis. Here is the recipe that I have found effective:

Air Passages: Alternative Approaches:

>1 cup sterile warm water
>1 tsp organic sea salt
>1 tsp baking soda
>1 tsp hydrogen peroxide (3%)
>5 drops organic eucalyptus oil

Place this mixture into a sterilized nasal spray container, or simply pour some into your palm and snort it up. A neti pot (available at most health food stores) can also be used to deliver the mixture into your sinuses.

Decline Purgation

This is an old method of draining and removing mucous from the bronchiole tree of the lungs without the use of suction or other invasive procedures done at the hospital. Fortunately this can be done in the privacy of your own home because you will be coughing and leaking sputum and mucous that has been clogging your respiratory system. People with asthma and COPD have a tendency to over produce mucous, which if left unchecked, can restrict breathing unto itself, and create the conditions for infection. Make sure that you are properly hydrated (see water therapy) and have not eaten for at least 2 hours prior to starting this therapy. This therapy is best attempted first thing in the morning and at night before bed.

WARNING: if you are hypertensive, do not attempt this without consulting your doctor first.

You will need a table or bed that can be elevated 16 inches off the ground, and ask a family member to help to massage/ lightly thump the area that is to be drained. Lean your body over the bed sideways with your feet hooking the mattress on the one side. You should feel comfortable enough to breath and not have too much pressure on your ribs or upper abdominal area. A cup to catch the sputum is advised. Have the family member gently thump (percuss) the mid-back upwards toward the head in a slow progressive fashion to dislodge the mucous from the bronchiole tree. Do this for no more than five minutes at a time.

Thumping

Thumping is a name I give to a technique I discovered while taking a shower one evening. I was having one of those days when I wasn't having an asthma attack directly, but there was a constant "heaviness' in my chest and my breathing was labored. I had worked out using Taijiquan for about 30 minutes to elevate my body temperature and decided to take a shower before bed. I climbed into the shower and turned on the warm water, which felt wonderful on my back. The shower head was set to pinpoint and was angled so that the warm spray hit right below the C7 vertebrae, which is the first vertebrae to protrude below your neck when your head is bent forward. I felt an almost instant relief of the pressure in my lungs, and my chest became instantly relaxed. It felt so wonderful to breathe deeply again that I stayed there for as long as the hot water held out. Later, I would learn through my acupuncture studies, that this is a key acupuncture point to treat asthma.

A quick word about showering in general. Make sure that you alternate hot and cold water on your body, always beginning with warm or hot water. Yes, I know this will dry your skin, but the hot water will suppress the itch from eczema. Always finish with a cool or cold shower, as this will cool the outside of the skin and close the pores. Finally moisturize thoroughly. Also, if you are not using a water filtration system for all your household water, at least purchase a filter for your bath showerhead. Chlorine in steam vapor can trigger an asthma attack as well as cause other serious problems.

Later I found that if moist heat (you can use one of several moist heating pads available) or activity warms the chest area, and if you can stimulate the back area (thumping), relief would come from your difficulty in breathing. Experimenting on this same idea, I found that cupping your hand and gently "thumping" the area around C7 will break up a lot of the mucous stagnation in the lung tissue during an asthma attack. Getting someone else to do this

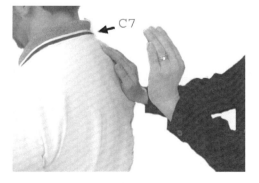

for you is a lot easier, trust me! Heat and thumping will not make the asthma attack go away, but they will offer some relief to the asthma patient by breaking up the thick, copious, sticky, phlegm that accompanies the asthma attack. The technique needs to be performed gently, with light taps to the back, and continuously (five to fifteen minutes) for best results.

One day, as I was doing volunteer work in a hospital, I went to pick up a patient in her room for physical therapy. I entered the room and noticed a man thumping the women's back in the same area that I had "discovered" in my thumping technique. I introduced myself and said that I would gladly wait until her "therapy" was completed. The man, who was a respiratory therapist performing the therapy, laughed and said " this is just a way to break up the mucous in her chest, so she can spit out some of the mucous to be analyzed by the doctors. Sure enough, she began to cough up phlegm and before long you could hear the phlegm breaking up inside of her lungs from her coughing, and then her breathing pattern changed to a more regulated, deeper breath.

My Herbal Tincture

Developing the tincture I am about to describe was a long arduous process. It evolved from my interest in natural medicines and supplementation. The tincture is designed to supplement my own body with enough of the chemical precursors for my body to produce its own natural prednisone. The tincture also offers adrenal support because these glands are often overstimulated by medications and treatment plans. Because this tincture rebalances the body so that it can produce its own cortisol and because it re-energizes the adrenals, this formula also supports immune function. I designed this specifically for myself and for my male body but many men and women have benefited from this concoction.

This tincture has also enjoyed great success in the reduction of pain from prostate inflammation. Many people take it daily to avoid catching colds and flus as well as to increase their feeling of vitality. Clients have told me that it must help bolster their immune system because they never get sick once they have been taking my tincture for a while.

The Latin names are listed here for accuracy, as many herbals have different compounds in them even though they may have the same common name. The primary ingredients are Medicago Sativa, Echinacea Angustifolia, Panax Ginseng, Centella Asiatica, Glycyrrhiza Glabra, Seronoa Repens, Dioscrea Oposita, Turnera Diffusa, Smilax Aristolochiaefolia in a mixture of alcohol and water.

Medicago Sativa. Alfalfa, sometimes called the "Father of all Foods" was discovered by the Arabs. In Chinese Medicine, this plant is used to treat digestive problems, particularly ulcers. It is also used to treat the infirm by stabilizing appetite. Ayurvedic medicine also uses it to treat fluid retention and arthritis pain. Alfalfa is an excellent source of most vitamins, especially A, D, E, and K and of the trace minerals of calcium, magnesium, iron, phosphorous and potassium. It also has the potential to neutralize acidic pH levels, balancing them out to alkaline.

Echinacea Angustifolia. The American Indians used this herb to treat everything from snakebite to influenza and colds. It has an antiviral, antifungal, and antibacterial properties, and is currently used in AIDS therapy. It stimulates white blood cells and is good for bolstering the immune system and the lymphatic system.

Panax Ginseng. All Ginsengs are not created equal; each variety has a slightly different action on the body. This herb is called Ren Shen in Chinese and is one of the most prized and expensive herbs. Classically known as a Yang tonic (more on this in chapter 14), it replenishes Qi or vital force to the Lungs and Spleen. In Chinese medicine, the Lungs and Spleen are usually compromised in allergies and asthma. In western medicine it has been shown to strengthen the immune system and decrease fatigue. Modern research has shown panax ginseng to be close to human sex hormones.

Centella Asiatica. This herb is a restorative for the nervous system as well as calming and relaxing.

Glycyrrhiza Glabra. This is the European species of licorice, but I have used the Chinese version with success as well. In China, this herb (Uralensis or Gan Cao) is called the great detoxifier and is thought to drive poisons from the system. It is often called the "grandfather of herbs." The root is used for gastric inflammation and as an anti-inflammatory for allergic conditions because it encourages adrenal function to return to normal after steroid therapy. It is used also to stimulate the lungs to expectorate by increasing the fluidity of mucus in the bronchial tubes. Avoid this herb if you have high blood pressure.

Seronoa Repens. Saw palmetto is called the "plant catheter" for its use in regulating and nutritionally benefitting the bladder and prostate in men. The berries have been used to treat diseases that rob the body of strength and growth, including thyroid deficiency. It is also excellent for clearing phlegm from the chest caused by asthma and bronchitis and it relieves cough.

Dioscrea Opposita. This particular yam has been used as a starter material to produce hydrocortisones for over the counter eczema creams. Called Shan Yao by the Chinese, it is used as a tonic herb to strengthen the Lungs, Stomach and Kidneys which according to Chinese Medicine theory, are often weak in asthmatics.

Dioscrea Villosa. (can be added additionally) Wild Yam has been used for centuries as a medicinal herb by the Aztec and Mayan peoples for a wide range of ailments, including gynecological problems and childbirth pain and inflammation. Research indicates that this is a powerful alternative medicine containing many steroidal saponins, mainly Dioscin which is widely used to manufacture progesterone and other steroid drugs used as contraceptives and in the treatment of various disorders of the genital organs as well as in other diseases such as asthma and arthritis. Other ingredients, including Phytosterols (beta-sitosterol), alkaloids and tannins, make this plant useful as an anti-inflammatory, antispasmodic, diaphoretic and vasodilator. Wild Yam is also used to treat irritable bowel syndrome (IBS), gastritis, gall bladder complaints, spasmodic cramps, painful menstruation, and, in small doses, is especially helpful in treating the nausea of pregnant women.

Turnera Diffusa. This is an excellent strengthening remedy for the nervous system and is especially soothing to the mucous membranes of the respiratory tract. It also has a famous reputation as a Yang tonic which regulates Qi stagnation in the stomach. In Chinese Medicine it is classically assigned for exhaustion, to relieve headaches and nervous debility, and to balance the hormones.

Smilax Aristolochiaefolia. Smilax has a reputation as a blood purifier and clinically was shown in 1942 to dramatically improve psoriasis. In the 1950's, it was shown to have antibiotic properties and used in human trials to treat leprosy. In homeopathy, it is used to treat itching. It has classic uses to stimulate metabolism and enhance glandular balance.

The secret of my herbal formula is combining the right amount of Yin and Yang properties in the selection of herbs. Each herb has its own properties that give its distinctive attributes. During the curing process the mixture must be exposed to the right amount of Yin (the moon) and Yang (the Sun). The electromagnetic forces of the earth affect the plants, much like the moon affects the tides. You might think this is odd, but to a person like me who grew up on a farm and was exposed to books like the Farmers Almanac, which still lists the best time to plant crops according to the moon phases, this is quite normal.

I generally like to make tinctures for myself. I believe that more of the essence of the plants is gathered by curing the plant for several weeks in alcohol (preferably grain alcohol as it is the most pure) than by any other means. I also like to take herbal tinctures sublingually (under the tongue) because the tincture enters my blood stream directly through the capillary beds in the mouth, bypassing the destructive enzymes and acids of the stomach. Once it hits the vat of acid in the stomach, the properties of the plant are chemically changed.

The craft and skill of creating custom tinctures is rapidly being lost with automation. I had the pleasure of working with a naturopathic doctor (ND) who was also a medical doctor (MD) he taught me how to bring the correct properties and balance to the mixture. If you can, see a naturopathic doctor, Chinese herbalists or others who have lived and loved herbals all his/her life and have that practitioner personally prepare something for your individual symptoms. This is preferable to buying a generic brand over the counter for something as important as your breathing and health.

(1) Serinus, Jason ed Psychoimmunity & the Healing Process Berkeley: Celestial Arts, 1986
(2) Wittenburg, Janice Strubbe, The Rebellious Body: Reclaim Your Life From Environmental Illness or Chronic fatigue , New York; Insight Books, 1996

CHAPTER 9

Stress

If there is one topic that we hear of more and more these days, it is stress and its adverse affects on health. For the asthmatic, it can be particularly devastating to one's health. *Stress can cause asthma attacks, and increase their duration, as well as exacerbate their intensity !*

We often hear the term "stressed out" or "stressed to the max", but what does that mean in terms of the body? Stress has another name, the "flight or fight mode." One could also add fright to this response mechanism. Whether an event is rational (example: fear) or imagined (example: anxiety), if we perceive that event as a threat or danger to our physical, emotional or spiritual self, we will kick the flight, fright or fight mode into gear. This has been known since the 1930's when Hanz Selye researched and predicted this pattern which he called general adaptation syndrome.

To illustrate how effectively the mind can control the body and bring on the fight or flight response, remember the last time you had a terrifying nightmare or vivid dream. The scenario could be a person chasing you with a long knife like in the horror movies or a situation where someone could be taking you to court for personal liability, for a divorce, or even a child custody battle. Serious situations for sure, ones where serious physical harm might happen or, at other extreme, prolonged mental anguish; but either can move you into the flight, fright or fight response or to use the catch all phrase...stress.

Let's examine what happens "when you don't sleep well." Although you were technically in your bed asleep with very limited physical movement at best, your body went through enormous chemical and physical reaction to "your thoughts." Sometimes you even scare yourself awake at which time you may notice how fast, heavily and deeply you are breathing and how quickly your heart is pounding in your chest. I have spoken with people who have awakened sweating from the intense activities of their "thoughts". You may even be exhausted from your sleep! Many people under duress from work experience this because they "are working" all night long trying to solve problems. This is a perfect example of how the perception of an event can reproduce the exact same physical reaction's as a real one.

Stress causes over 1,500 different chemical reactions in the body per stressful event! That means that each time you go into flight, fright or fight mode, you literally become a pharmaceutical dump of various chemicals that react in the body. Some of these very chemicals can be the cause of skin eruptions, immune system disorders and triggers for asthma attacks.

The fight, fright or flight response was designed to protect and preserve us in case of danger. Some of the responses of the body produced by this self-preservation mechanism are as follows. (This may get a little technical but you will see how it all ties in together in the following pages.)

The pupils of the eyes dilate to allow more light in for more accurate vision in the dark to escape danger or to fight. Adrenal hormone production increases to allow increased respiration; blood pressure goes up in order to pump more oxygen through the blood to the muscles and brain for enhanced response time. The adrenal cortex produces steroid hormones, including hydrocortisone, cortisone, testosterone, estrogen, 17-hydrooxyketosteroids, DHEA, pregnenolone, aldosterone, androstenedione, and progesterone! What a list! Your body goes into this chemical overtime production upon command from your mind. You may recognize these chemicals from articles on hormone replacement therapy, or on their use in sports performance.

Adrenal Burnout

Aldosterone works with the renal system (the kidneys) to regulate sodium and potassium levels in the body. If unregulated, a person may develop further irregular adaptations to fight, fright or flight, such as irregular blood pressure with a common symptom of puffy hands and feet. Recent western medical experiments have shown that one can have adrenal fatigue, or adrenocortical disease, without adrenal function failure. [1]

This research may dismay allopathic doctors, who for years claimed that alternative practitioners who treat for adrenal burnout brought about through long-term stress were incapable of showing any clinical proof.

Through the release of catecholamines, the liver releases glucose or blood sugar (gluconeogenesis) which has been stockpiled away for emergencies, as when the brain and the muscles make extra demand for flight or fight. The brain demands its blood sugar first, before any muscle even 'thinks' about getting blood sugar. The stress response also triggers the pulling of blood away from the extremities of the body, so that if cut, scratched or hit, the body will not lose as much blood or bruise as badly. Movement of blood to areas of the body needed for fighting and running also takes blood from areas of the body; like the digestive tract; which are not necessary for the immediate task. Therefore, if you are eating lunch after a stressful meeting with your boss or are upset before lunch for any reason, you may want to use some of the QiGong and meditation techniques discussed later in the book before eating. Otherwise, what will happen is the food that you eat will be digested, but the transportation mechanism (the blood) will not be there to deliver the nutrients elsewhere, so it just stays put. No nutrition is delivered, you get an upset stomach, and you still have not taken care of the root of the problem! If you or a loved one suffer from irritable bowel, Crohn's disease or are constantly taking antacids, check your stress levels. When we talk about what happens to someone in athletic competition or in a life-threatening situation, we use the phrase, "his adrenaline was pumping". Yes, this is true, but so much more is happening than we realize. All these automatic responses take place in a matter of seconds and can continue in this mode for a reasonable period of time.

In fact, one of the stress hormones that we commonly know as adrenaline may stimulate the growth of bacteria in the body. This may be why people always seem to come down with a cold or flu after they have been under great periods of stress. In addition, the stress hormones norepinephrine and epinephrine can suppress certain components of the immune system. [2]

When you have been on edge for several days, take notice, as I have, how your throat feels, if your mucous production picks up, and if you feel unnaturally tired! For someone with asthma, this can be another factor that creates the potential for asthma attack. We already know that stress affects the immune system through high cortisol concentrations and lowered DHEA, scientists do not know the point at which these changes begin to do damage. Adrenal hyperfunction, makes the body more susceptible to insulin resistance, hypertension, mild obesity, and elevated serum levels of triglycerides and lipids (cholesterol). In the final stages of long-term stress, the body is unable to regulate its cortisol levels and other corticosteroids hormones levels. This can lead to excessive fatigue, inability to concentrate, menstrual irregularities, hypoglycemia, and weight gain through carbohydrate sensitivity. The body loses its ability to control inflammation, key to the asthmatic and allergy sufferer, and the body goes into a pro-inflammatory state leading to tissue damage and further degenerative disease.

Managing Your Stress

I am willing to bet that in the future asthmatics will resort to stress management courses as a way to help control their asthma; perhaps insurance companies even will pay for the courses as part of preventative medicine.

The thing to remember is that stress - or flight, fright or fight - was designed to be a brief encounter. The life-style we live today, from the stressful ride into work in the morning to feeling like you're falling behind on your deadlines, is a constant drain on your body's reserves and your immunity. The body was never designed to endure stress from the time you wake up until the time you collapse on the couch at the end of the day. Chronic stress places your body at potential risk for a whole host of health risks, from heart attack to a decrease in immune function which can lead to such diseases as chronic fatigue syndrome, irritable bowel syndrome (IBS), ulcers, asthma attacks and eczema flare-ups.

Additionally, stress can also cause us to have a mental block or to forget something that we know quite well. Forgetting peoples names, directions to a local store, even our medication that we have taken for years, can all be blamed on stress forgetfulness. During a test, were you ever unable to remember an answer even though you can "see the page" of the book you studied? Then, as soon as the test is over and you relax, the answer comes to you plain as day.

Your stress is entirely yours and no one gave it to you, as we often hear. I do mean that literally in the sense that it is entirely yours in your own mind. Many times, what stresses you can not be seen or understood by anyone but you. How your mind works and perceives, evaluates facts and events, and pieces stories together is unique to you and only you. Our own self-talk is a curious thing. Often we don't even speak our thoughts exactly to ourselves or others. We rephrase them. We all do this; as it is perfectly normal. The point is that our internal dialog is a manifestation of our own unique combination of biology, environment, coping skills and tools, and our own one-of-a-kind mindfulness that gives us our individuality.

In fact, many times it is the lack of perception of what's stressing you that is the cause of many arguments, disagreements, and the lack of communication between two parties. Have you ever been in a bad mood when someone asks you an innocent question that sends you into a tirade? Your mindset and your coping skills (or lack thereof) can cause misunderstandings between two people very quickly. Your perceptions of what is stressful begin and end in your own mind. Not being able to say what is bothering you, or not being able to verbalize this to another person, can cause a rift of understanding between two parties.

The game plan to combat stress includes many lifestyle changes as well as certain compromises of body and mind (effective change requires compromise). Gaining better control over your stress depends on how effectively you want to combat this problem and therefore your degree of commitment. To totally reduce stress from our lives would be an accomplishment that involves a spiritual transition that is beyond the scope of this book. Stress and total peace are at the opposite ends of the continuum, and everyone has to decide at what point on that continuum they will be satisfied to live their lives.

Effective stress management requires a multilevel, multidimensional program. Understand that the beginning levels of this stress program are easier to accomplish, but also have less long-term effect in overall stress reduction. In other words, you get out what you put in. The changes in order of easiest to most difficult are as follows:

Physical changes: These include eating intervals, rest and sleep intervals, time management skills, and programmed body movement intervals (structured physical exercises).

Relaxation changes: More difficult to obtain but more effective these relaxation changes are about the relaxation and clearing the mind of clutter and include: visualization, meditation, breathing patterns, mantras and projection of the positive self.

Spiritual changes: The last stage, a stage beyond the scope of this book, is about spiritual training and a change to the highest plane.

Let us begin our stress management program with the easiest changes to adapt to, the changes of the physical kind.

Chronobiology

Everything that is living goes through rhythms or cycles. Even Mother Earth has rhythms and cycles, from the tides of the oceans to the rise and fall of the Sun. Everything oscillates at a certain tempo. As human beings, most of us have learned to coexist with these natural rhythms to enhance and sustain life. However, every once in a while we start to believe that we can reinvent nature and stop abiding by its rules. That is where we start to get in trouble so far as our health is concerned.

The Chinese have studied the cycles of men and women in accordance with nature for thousands of years. Governed in empirical observation, their common sense wisdom has been well documented, but only recently have their insights been proven scientifically through the new emerging science call chronobiology. Chronobiology is the study of biological rhythms and how they relate to exercise, the body's ability to burn calories, sleep, sex and healing. Chronotherapy is the use of the natural body rhythms of the human body to enhance one's ability, for instance, to better absorb prescription medications, so that less dosage is required. From the western medical perspective, we know that blood testosterone levels peak at 8-9pm and that the level of glucocorticoid tapers throughout the daylight hours, beginning to rise around 4am and peaking at 6-8 am. For asthmatics, the respiratory system reaches its peak of airway resistance around 5 am, coinciding with nighttime asthma and the simultaneous drop of glucocorticoid.

Chronotherapy has been in use for thousands of years in the Chinese Medical system, and in many cases serves as the foundation of treatment protocol, especially in Medical QiGong therapy (more on this later in chapter 14). The following diagram shows the natural human cycles (the Tao) according to Chinese energetic theory based on our 24 hour clock.

Air Passages: Stress

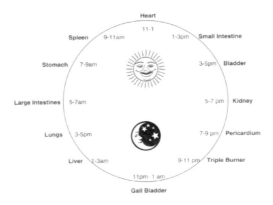

Let us start with the work/rest cycle. For every given period of work, there should be a period of rest. This statement makes enough sense to us that it should almost go without saying. However, think about what happens to us in the workplace with deadlines, climbing the corporate ladder, down-sizing and doing the work of two people, and our own personal agenda. We push the limits of endurance.

We would easily understand the work/rest cycle if we were to continuously swing an eight pound sledgehammer without stopping for an hour. We would need to take a rest. However, somehow we have concluded that we can push our minds to operate at top performance hour after hour, day after day, without any rest. The rest here that I am speaking of is in the form of play, relaxation and diversion. Remember how you used to play as a child? Remember that you used to tell your Mom you were bored? When is the last time that you said that you had extra time on your hands and were bored? A child laughs 600 times per day. How often as an adult do you laugh per day?

For every 90 minutes of mindful intense thinking or concentrating, try to take at least 10 to 15 minutes of rest. This rest period can be accomplished by just getting up from your desk and chair and stretching a few minutes (see the exercise chapter) or by looking at the vacation picture on your desk and thinking about the great time you had there. To change your scenery, take a walk outside, down the hall, or anywhere. We will naturally change our scenery by daydreaming, if we do not schedule these breaks into our day. We have all caught ourselves daydreaming or fantasizing. Daydreaming is a pressure release valve that operates in the body if we do not consciously take heed of our natural cycles. Take some time to play. Buy a comic book, climb a tree, do anything that is reminiscent of being in your youth when the school days took forever. Learn to play again.

Along with changing scenery, you need to refuel the brain. The brain is a glucose or blood sugar hog and can consume twice the amount of blood sugar during intense thinking as during rest. So, if you are problem solving or being creative at work or at home with the kids, you need to have your blood sugar fueling your brain cells. Now let me preface this by saying that you do not have to have a banquet every 90 minutes! A small piece of complex carbohydrate is all you need, just a bite or two. Somehow, in America we think that we have to have a meal every time we sit down to eat, as if size and quantity is everything!

Here are some of the better foods for people with allergies to keep handy at work or at school to sustain them during heavy periods of mental activity.

- Angel food cake
- Apples
- Cherries
- Dark rye bread
- Dried apricots
- Dried bananas
- Melba toast
- Oatmeal cookies
- Rice cakes
- Yogurt

Time Management

When it comes to managing time, we all have our own theories. However, prioritizing what is important is one of the fundamentals of good time-management skills. Keep an itinerary, whether you use a Palm pilot, a Daytimer, or a folded up piece of paper with your today's events on it. Keep it with you always; write down ideas, moments of enlightenment that you will want to remember later. Leonardo DaVinci, one of the greatest thinkers and inventors who ever existed, was way ahead of his time in many ways. He always carried with him a piece of paper and pencil to scribble down ideas. We can emulate him by prioritizing what tasks we want to get accomplished each day and writing them down in the order of importance. Things like "twenty minutes to exercise," "10 minutes to pray," an "hour to play with the kids or the spouse," a "half-hour to read or study," all need to be written down and allocated in your busy day. Otherwise these things are cast aside and we wonder, "where did the time go?" Perhaps you say to yourself, "I wished I would have spent more time with my grandmother, mother, sister, dog, or my children. I wish I had spent time volunteering for a worthy cause". All of the truly important events can magically get replaced by other things to do. What really is important in your life? Write it down, schedule it for yourself and control your life. Don't just try to "fit it in." Suzie Ormond, the financial genius who always says, "pay yourself first" has the right idea, only schedule time to play first. Life is too short.

I really do subscribe to ideas in Steven Covey's book <u>The 7 Habits of Highly Effective People</u> and I think that reading that book should be high on your list of things to do. The other important thing as you keep your list and prioritize the items on it, is to enjoy crossing them off. You can now chart your progress of getting things accomplished and feel good about it. Basic, simple stuff, I know, but like anything else in life, the basics always work best and always better than elaborate schemes. Concentrate on the basics first. Make your life about basics and fundamentals.

I have already given enough information on programmed movement or exercise. It does have to be programmed into a part of your daily schedule. A good rule of thumb is that the body needs to move and stretch fully every two hours. You change positions in your sleep about that often as the brain wave frequency changes from the four levels of sleep (S1 through S4). These four levels cycle every 90 minutes leading to the REM (rapid eye movement) state. Think about driving for several hours. Usually about the second hour your body signals you to change positions, go to the bathroom, or get a drink, all things designed to make you move.

From the physical, to the chemical, to the psychological, to the social, stress probably does more to affect us in our everyday lives than any other factor. Knowing how to get a handle on stress, and become its master, rather than let it dominate us, is the topic of our next chapter, controlling the mind, which is also the second level. Remember that the stress response is being elicited in our brain by our own mind from own perceptions, self talk, or your version of reality.

(1) Subclinical Cushing's Syndrome in adrenal incidentaloma. Clinical Endocrinal 19998;48(1):89-97.
(2) WebMD Medical News May 25, 2000.

CHAPTER 10

The Mind

"The final mystery is oneself....

who can calculate the orbit of his own soul"

Oscar Wilde

This chapter is probably the most important part of this book. This is the chapter where I will describe the one thing that probably saved my life more times than any other medical treatment that I have ever encountered. This chapter is about gaining control of your body through the use of your mind. This is first accomplished by using tools most people refer to as meditation.

The mind/body link has been widely talked about in America by the general public since the 60's; but this talk has often been tentative or reserved. Most people agree that the mind has something to do with the body's healing, or lack of. We understand that in athletic performance that concentration, attitude, confidence, and all those other things we somehow manage to lump together as "the mind" are important in separating victory from defeat, success from failure, and survival from extinction.

What we don't know, however, are the details of how the mind works or even why it works and why sometimes it seems to fail us. To explain and understand the mind, we look to conventional Newtonian science to somehow come up with a linear, three dimensional, algorithmic explanation that can be replicated by anyone, as if we were playing a game of golf and these are the rules to play by. We look to scientists to explain something that they themselves have not dedicated their lives to understanding. We ask them to explain it to us, write it down in a textbook, and then teach a class on it. How far, despite all of our knowledge, we have strayed from the simple truth of life is amazing. If we are to learn how to use our mind to its fullest degree, then we should study those who have dedicated their lives to the practice of the mind and its teachings.

There is a Zen saying, "The ancient teachings illuminate the mind and the mind illuminates the ancient teachings." Most ancient indigenous cultures had gurus, priests, sages and masters who made the journey toward inner peace, calmness, and becoming one with the universe the focus of their very existence. Some cultures that are over several thousand years old such as Chinese, Indian and the Hopi Indians, continue this line of thinking. If you would talk to people who have (by the declaration of their peers rather than themselves) mastered their minds they would tell you that they only scratched the surface in their search for how the mind works, for how it is unified, for how it can unlock untold peace and happiness. And yes, it can also heal the body. The amazing thing is that these sages do not care in the least why or how it works (the reductionism approach), just that it does and that is enough for them. This faith is the beginning of the journey. Because there is only so much sand in the hourglass, there is only so much time to experience those grains; you choose how you want to utilize those grains of time.

Jalaluddin Rumi said, "The true teacher knocks down the idol that the student makes of him." The enlightened masters (if I dare call them that), all admit that the journey has only begun for them and they eagerly await the next piece of progress that they can make. When these same masters try to explain why a person would want to invest the dedication, persistence and desire necessary to pursue the activities of the mind, many people can't hear the masters. They think that only their "to-do" list as worthy enough of their time and energies. How sad. The very people who need it the most miss the message. It is not my point to try to convert anyone to spending time in meditation or dedicating their lives to its study, but let me also be clear that those who don't consider the mind an important element in the healing process are in grave error, regardless of how much they think they know or what level of education they have.

Sometimes we think we never have enough information to make decisions, so we actively pursue more education, more data on the Internet, more books to read, or we study with this person and that person. The real answer, however, is to sit and be still, to meditate if you will. All that you have and have been given, all that makes you the microcosm of who and what you are, will create the innate ability to arrive at answers for yourself. This is the greatest secret of the ancients.

However, in our society, where we are driven to obtain and retain more information more and more quickly to maintain the edge over the competition. The fact is, we are moving further from the basic truths than ever before in history. We push ourselves to move and produce even when we are fatigued. The only time we finally sit in silence is when we are too tired to say anything let alone have energy to concentrate. When was the last time that you sat in silence with your partner, your children and/or your parents, in a loving enjoyable quiet solitude that was so nurturing and comfortable? We are taught that in order to be having a good time we must be talking, laughing, partying and carrying on. I think some of the most precious times are the ones spent in silence with the ones you love and who love you. The quite time to sit and be still, not just with yourself, but also with your spouse, your mother and father, your children or even your pet, is such a precious thing. The connection we make at that level of relaxation is something we all strive for and relish, yet we can't seem to see this simple solution.

This is the beginning of understanding true knowledge and empowerment. The idea of "relaxing by doing" must be the greatest lie of the 20th century and beyond. I see people on vacation who measure the quality of a good time by how much they did and saw. I see them on their vacation, teaching their children the exact same message by example: that we must hurry, rush, cram it all in, so that we can rush back to work the following day into the same hectic lifestyle that we were desperately trying to escape. The nuclear family concept of relaxation is to "get away from it all" and "rest." This constant adrenaline rush to accomplish and finish, to get done and move on, to place another notch in the belt, drains the very core of our body of vital energy. Our poor adrenal glands responding to our mental process (yes, this is the stress response of fight or flight too) have unprecedented demands placed upon them. I suspect that adrenal burnout is the foundation of most illness and disease in the industrialized nations. From the alarm clock scaring us out of our sleep, to getting the kids ready and off to daycare on time, to battling the traffic and construction delays on the highways (not to mention all the "idiots" on the road), you have the making of a combat zone of adrenal failure in your first two hours of waking!

But how do we begin to change our intent and commit to what is meaningful to us? Again, by doing the most simple and basic things. But given our upbringing and habits of mind, including how we were taught to learn, we must use tools to help us. The first of the tools that I enjoyed as a child was meditation. After we examine meditation, we will explore other tools, such as guided visualization and the highest level of mind cultivation called Qigong.

Meditation

There is a tale told by the ancient Greeks, who metaphorically used the discussion of Gods to teach the lessons of life. The Gods on Mount Olympus were having a discussion about their greatest project to date …mankind. They had already created all living things in perfect balance (Yin and Yang) and were discussing the most difficult of decisions…..where to hide the secret of life for humans. The hiding place could not be anyplace where someone could just stumble upon the treasure. It had to be a place reached only after a long journey of dedication, persistence and sacrifice. The seekers consciousness must evolve on the journey so that when the seeker did find this great knowledge, the seeker would not abuse the power it contains. The first God said, "Let us hide it in the tallest most forbidding mountain as man will never find it there." Another God spoke up quickly and stated emphatically that "We have created man with an insatiable curiosity and ambition, and he will eventually climb even the highest mountain." A God across the room said, "Then we will hide it in the deepest trench of the sea". To which another replied, "Man has boundless imagination and a burning desire to explore his world. Sooner or later this place too would be discovered." Finally, one of the elder Gods spoke and said, "Let us hide the secret of life in the last place that man would ever look." The other Gods grew silent for a moment and then asked, "And where might that be"? To which the elder God replied, "Deep in the heart of man."

It is interesting to note that in Chinese Medicine, the Shen, or the Spirit, is said to reside in the heart as well. Maybe the ancients knew something? Ah, but now the question still remains ….how to get to that place in modern times.

Meditation is stillness, being alive in the great void where all things become possible; a one point of focus joined with ten-thousand unions. Meditation puts you in a state of peace and calm, but not, as many people think solitude. The higher levels of meditation bring an intuitive, intrinsic feeling of joining with something much greater than ourselves. After spending over 30 years researching various disciplines for the "secret one" meditation that was going to save and cure me, I finally concluded that the following processes work best for me and people like me.

I think most of us want to know before we commit to something, what rewards we can expect with persistent and dedication to my practice. What can I gain from meditation? The following are all things I encounter as by-products of my original intent. I am still learning, improving and growing and will continue to, but I definitely feel that meditation has helped me in the following areas.

Meditation allows me to focus and concentrate better. This is probably the greatest gift for someone who has to work for a living….namely all of us. Being efficient enough to perform a number of tasks in a short period of time is essential in today's hectic, fast-paced world. Meditation helps us to focus better on work tasks as well as on the "to-do" list at home and with family. Taking time to meditate will help you make better use of your time because of your ability to think in a sharper, clearer and more intense way.

Has this ever happened to you? You are trying to troubleshoot something at work or around the house, and just cannot seem to find a solution. You instinctively know that it shouldn't be this hard, but you just can't solve the puzzle. Then as you wake up the next morning, or in your dreams at night, you miraculously "discover" the answer. The answer was always there, but you just could not retrieve it when needed. Another example that you might relate to; the taking of college or high school tests. Think of all the times you've taken a test in school and just couldn't remember the answer, but as soon as you handed in your test, walked down the hall and had a drink, the answer comes to you. Stress and anxiety do this to you; they make you forget the things that you have recently learned.

Muscular tension is probably something you have noticed when you are "having one of those days." You instinctively grab the back of your neck and massage it with your hand, lifting your head up as you do. Ah, the infamous tension headache is on its way. Again, a product of stress.

Meditation can help in the following ways:

1. Relieve stress, anxiety, and muscular tension
2. Clear your thinking and enhance your creativity
3. Lower blood pressure and cholesterol

4. Overcoming addictive behaviors or negative self talk
5. Increase your self-awareness
6. Obtaining more happiness and enjoyment from simple activities
7. Deepen the sense of meaning in your life

And for those of you who need scientific evidence, researcher Dr. Andrew Newberg of the University of Pennsylvania School of Medicine reported that a number of areas of the brain respond to meditation in a number of areas in the brain. Using this research, let's take the example of meditating at a mountain lake in the fall. As you begin to concentrate on nature's beauty, the frontal lobe that controls motivation is activated. As you observe the wind blowing through the trees, the motion activates the temporal lobe which processes visual stimuli when you focus on the slight ripples of the lake. The feeling of awe or joy stemming from the beauty of nature also invigorates the temporal lobe. As you start to go into the zone of meditation or feel as if "everything's connected," the processing sensations at the top part of the parietal lobe begin to calm down. Dr. Newberg's research also shows meditation can be documented as having a calming effect on the mind as well as the body.

Having a calm day is almost unheard of in our culture. Most professional Americans I know are very concerned with time and wasting it. We are so frenzied in our typical days that we cannot perceive anything that does not give immediate gratification and reward. Anything else is "a waste of time". Meditation, even if coached correctly from the first lesson, is a long journey. Prepare for that. One of the interesting paradoxes I find in working with people is that the people who need meditation the most "don't have time to do it."

Meditation has been around as long as man has chosen to sit quietly and relax. Whether through prayer, trancing, visualizing, drumming or entering an altered state through herbal preparations, man has always longed for tranquility and for connection with a "higher power". One will lead to the other because they are both the same.

It does take persistence and tenacity to approach the point where you can truly reap the benefits of these practices. This is why someone who is plagued by illness or suffering may be somewhat more successful than others using meditation. This group of people has so much more to gain than any other group, with far less to lose (like time invested). A healthy business executive, told that "meditation is good for your health and you should practice this every day" would probably say, even if they were interested, "I just don't have time." But if that same executive has heart disease, with a family history of premature death from stroke or heart attack; or their triglycerides and cholesterol levels are through the roof;, or two blocked carotid arteries leading to their brain, she/he might start to see the value of meditation as a means to de-stress.

Ask anyone who had a frightening illness or has been diagnosed with a terminal illness what one thing is most important in life. Here is a hint: it is not money. It is your health. To regain your health is worth every minute of time invested and even every dollar of your hard earned money in order to be coached correctly. If this were not true, Americans would not be spending billions of dollars on alternative health care. I think the most important point here is to be proactive in your disease. Do not let the disease control you and your mind (depression, anxiety, etc.), but take control again by trying something. Even if it means you do not get the intended miraculous result, you have not failed and the modality has not failed. This may not be the right modality of treatment for you, but it may work well for someone else. Keep trying. Do not allow yourself to be mentally beaten up by lack of desired immediate results.

I think an overlooked step to successfully doing what I call Visualization Meditation Techniques (VMT) is to understand what you are trying to visualize. I learn more quickly using visuals; I must see pictures in my mind for me to feel comfortable with concepts or ideas. This is the same way I approached my VMT's. I was always interested in the human body. What a magnificent, extraordinary, computerized machine it is. As a teenager, I bought books on anatomy and physiology and read them, like most people read a novels. Naturally, I was fascinated by how the lungs worked, or in my case why they didn't work well. I was intrigued to find out how the alveoli (little sacs that exchange gases between the lungs and the blood) remain inflated during an asthma attack and do not let any more air in. I even found out that there are special cells called alveolar macrophages, that devour dust particles from the alveolar. The human body designed a cell to vacuum up its own dust and dispose of it! Now that is recycling at its best. I devoured the details of how the lung looked and functioned and then tried to feel them working as I went on my day-to-day tasks.

I then used this information to make my VMT's more real to me. When I meditated, I knew what I was talking and thinking about with clear concise pictures in my mind. To effectively combat asthma or any illness, you must first have all the facts and details (at least what knowledge is known at that time) in order for you to have a combat strategy.

When I worked as a personal trainer, one of the most common complaints I heard was "I can't relax," "I'm too stressed out," or "It takes two days on vacation before I can decompress enough to start to enjoy myself." How sad. Other versions of this problem are having to "unwind" before going to sleep or having to watch TV to "take their mind off things".

Although everyone's lifestyle is complicated, hectic and demanding these days, some of the anxiety could be eradicated by taking a few moments to deep breathe, visualize, and relax naturally. I realize finding a few minutes to yourself is probably rare, especially if you have younger children. But, a reality check: you probably spend 20 to 40 minutes either watching television, tossing or turning, or lying awake anyway. Why not give yourself 10 minutes before you go to bed to program your mind for pleasant dreams, restful sleep. Save yourself time and frustration by getting the rest your body so desperately needs.

There are three phases that I will walk you through on your journey to using VMT's. They are Visualization, Breathing methods and Healing meditations. Try to repeat these steps every day at whatever time of the day is best for you based on your asthma and time availability. After three months of doing this routine, increase the visualization and breathing to twice per day. After six months, increase again the visualizations/breathing to three times per day. I realize that this is a chunk of time, but it is necessary to develop the lungs and the adaptive process of your body slowly.

Visualization

The human mind has over 60,000 thoughts per day. With all of that work going on, wouldn't you want to control at least part of this huge deliberation with something positive? The first step, visualization, is the easiest. You may want to read this next exercise session into a cassette or CD to play back as if someone is coaching you in the room. This will be easier than trying to remember all the fine points. This is a beginning exercise to allow you to gauge your visualization grade level. Some individuals may be able to envision all the pictorial changes right away, some will lose their concentration. Others will be able to do the exercise in its entirety, but not see it in 3D or in living color. It is important that the visualization be as real as the most vivid dream you can ever remember having. When you can do this, then you move on to breathing methods. It is more important to master these basic concepts in the beginning before you try to combine all phases of VMT's together.

The following exercise proved to be quite successful when I worked as a stress consultant for the Federal Governments Social Security Program in 1999. Participants loved it so much that I put this exercise on my Self Defense for Stress video.

In all visualization exercises you can either sit or stand. The important thing is to be comfortable. Have someone read this to you very slowly, allowing your mind time to "see, smell and taste" the description.

Sit back and relax. In your mind, see a large red delicious apple. Rotate the apple around in your mind and analyze the color, the slight imperfections. Notice the smoothness of the skin and how upon closer examination, the apple skin actually isn't all red but has flecks of white intermixed with the red. Rotate the apple again and examine the bottom of the apple. Notice the four large dimples surrounding the bottom part of the core. Notice the symmetry of the corners. Now rotate the apple again to the top. See the brown stem sticking out from the middle. Notice two large green leaves also attached to the stem.

Now place the apple on a hard surface and with one blow of a very sharp knife, cut the apple into two pieces. Examine the white flesh of the apple; notice the juice running from the flesh of the apple and over the red skin. Can you smell the apple juice? Now take the same knife and cut the two halves into quarters. Again, notice the pure white flesh contrasting the redness of the skin. On one of the quarters, is the stem sticking out from the top? Now, we will start to reassemble the apple. Bring the quarters back together into perfect, crisp halves. Now bring the two halves together forming the uniform, unblemished apple that you originally started with. Open your eyes.

How long did you think this exercise took?

Actually in the mind, there is no such thing as time. Time is distorted by your intense concentration and the relaxation response. This same concept operates in daydreaming. The scariest form of daydreaming is catching yourself at work and wondering how long you were like that, and more importantly, if anyone noticed! Of course we all daydream, but next time you catch yourself, see if you can figure out how long you were in the "zone."

Visualization actually starts in the higher centers of the brain (the cerebral cortex) and filters to lower sections of the brain (the limbic system) that control breathing, heart rate, blood flow and blood pressure, digestion and the immune response.

The limbic system is what allows us to learn and rehabilitate from injury and trauma and is vastly important in sports medicine and learning new skills. Within the brainstem is an area called the reticular activating system (RAS) that is responsible for the transmission of learning to the cerebral cortex. Visualization and meditation use this loop of information supplied by nervous and electrical energy to allow us to maximize learning and remembering when in a relaxed state of being.

You can visualize any scene you choose. A beach, a favorite vacation spot, serene forest, Yellowstone National Park, anything that makes you feel relaxed and at peace.

Gradually in your visualization practice, you can make the scenes you "see" in the mind more complex. For healing purposes, you must work toward making your visuals more realistic to you. Most of us do this by adding more and more detail to the scene, thereby making it more believable to ourselves. This accumulation of detail is like what digital animation has done for movies, (think of the *Lord of the Rings* movies or *Shrek*). The more detail it has, the more we feel that the story is real. Again, it is not that we focus on the background, but the background makes us believe that what is happening is real. People who go to movies and cry, or feel the rush of adrenaline as the music begins to climb and intensify, are actually suspending their belief system for the duration of the movie. We know the movie is not "real," but we can elicit an emotional response from that set of events and "live" the moment through our suspension of belief. The more we cultivate the attention to detail and appeal to all five senses, the more we feel the authenticity of the set, whether in the movie theater or in visualization.

This intense focus and concentration must then be held steady in the mind for greater periods of time. Once you begin to acquire this ability, it will facilitate a physical response from the body in the form of total relaxation or, at the highest level, healing. One of my first martial arts masters would answer my questions (of which there were so many) by telling me, "The answers to your questions are all within you, but you must allow them to come to the surface". He would say, "First you must be able to hold a single thought in your mind for several minutes." I thought, how hard can that be? I was amazed by how much the human mind drifts into tangents of rapid, uninterrupted, incongruent, thoughts. Holding a single thought for a couple of seconds is tough, but for five, 10 or fifteen minutes was impossible, or so I told myself.

One day he placed a candle on the table and lit it. He asked me to sit down and face the candle. He said, "sit and be still, don't take your eyes off the candle. Allow the candle to be all that you see and all that you feel. Every time your mind wanders, focus on the candle flame and see the colors within it change. Bring your mind to a single purpose, a single thought and hold it there. Allow all the self-talk and dialogue that you have within yourself to cease and just concentrate on the flame." The exercise worked because it gave me something tangible to focus on, rather than closing my eyes and not knowing how to regulate my thoughts. A funny by-product of this training happened. As I became more advanced in my candle exercise, I noticed my free sparring and fighting skills improving dramatically.

Later, upon analyzing what was happening, I realized that I was able to relax my body although I was fighting. By doing so, I was able to move much more quickly and efficiently. In fact, I was able to "read" my opponent's intentions and movements before he was committed to the action. This allowed me an extra half a second to a full second to respond to his attack and to counter. I was able to outmaneuver my opponent not by becoming physically faster in technique, but by improving my timing and ability to respond through the relaxation response.

In the Japanese classic <u>The Book of Five Rings</u>, an aging samurai wrote down all of the tactics he would use in battle to remain undefeated. This book used to be applied to warfare, but now is applied to business management practices and is required reading in Japan for an MBA. In fact, to this day, negotiation with Japanese businessman remains one of the true tests for any American businessman. The book emphasizes learning to anticipate your "opponent's" move and therefore develop a strategy well in advance of your opponent's execution. This is done by the practice of visualization and calming of the mind.

Breathing Techniques for Guided Visualization

Once you have the ability to visualize and hold a thought for several minutes, it's time to start adding breathing methods to the mix. Actually, if you are performing the visualizations correctly, you probably are breathing at a much slower and more even pace than you normally do.

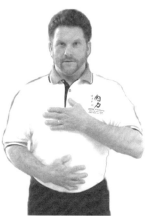

Let's try several experiments to see where you are in maximizing your genetic potential for deep breathing. Place one hand on your chest and another on your stomach above your belly button. Now just breathe normally. Which one moved? If the chest hand is moving, you are a chest breather. For the most part, you want to become a belly breather, in other words you want the hand on the stomach to move more than the hand on the chest.

Most people are not aware that when you belly breathe, you should not only feel the belly expand through diaphragmatic compression, but you should also feel the small of your back move as well. When the small of the back begins to move, the full expansion of the body is complete. Only then are you truly using the full capacity of your body to gather precious oxygen.

In America, we are so body conscious of our stomachs and our posture. We thrust our shoulders back and chest out when we walk, a way of moving that puts us in constant muscular contraction. This kind of posture does not allow the stomach to stick out as we inhale. Holding in the stomach actually facilitates chest breathing and uses muscles located near your ribs, called the intercostals, to perform the inhalations.

Air Passages: The Mind

To see a different kind of breath watch the chest and stomach of someone when who is asleep. We can always tell when someone falls into a deep sleep by their breathing patterns. Typically, the person's rhythm of breathing changes and so does the depth of their inhalations and exhalations. The diaphragm is now released from the muscular tension of being sucked in and the whole musculature of the upper body is allowed to relax and be natural. It is fine to have good posture and walk with purpose and pride, but not at the expense of our health.

Another test for illustrating correct breathing technique is to bend over at the waist and place your palms on the tops of your knees. Now just breathe normally. You will find that it is almost impossible to breathe "wrong" (ie..chest breathing) when in this position. You will see many people who sprint, run marathons, and even play football assume this position after a run in order to regain composure through proper breathing methods. In fact, I know of one music/ voice instructor who teaches this technique to his students to help them understand the concept of belly breathing.

Another interesting point was brought to my attention by one of my Kungfu students who happens to be a voice (singing) coach. He informed me that by breathing in with the mouth in an "ee" (long e) sound, you promote clavicular high breathing. Conversely, by breathing in with the mouth in a long "oooo" sound, you promote lower diaphragmatic breathing. Interestingly enough, the Taoist priest that I study with employs many different sounds to vibrate and work different parts of the body. It appears that many cultures and professions know about the secrets of breath and sounding!

Remember, when exercising or meditating you want the chest, stomach and lower back all to expand upon inhaling. This allows a greater tidal volume of air to come into the body and allows the body to tap into an endless supply of energy known as fat cells. You will actually burn fat much more efficiently when you exercise, if you learn to breathe correctly! Try to apply these new patterns to your exercise programs previously discussed.

Air Passages: The Mind

Healing Meditations

This section is very much based on my study of Chinese medicine and on various meditations I created for myself in my search for the Holy Grail for asthma. There is no such Holy Grail yet, but these meditations will take you to a deeper level of meditation than you ever thought possible.

I have used these meditations to save my life more than once. These meditations will lower your pulse rate and allow you to relax without muscular tension so that your medications can work more effectively. I have used these meditations to quiet my body and mind down until I could reach my medications when I stupidly forget my "rescue remedy" (Albuterol).

First, a short story and then the meditation. I will preface this story by saying that I had been so successful in managing my asthma for years, that I no longer focused on this being a problem for me. Thanks to nutrition, exercise and meditation management, carrying my "rescue remedy" with me at all times had slipped my mind. I am not proud of this day, but I share it with you to show the power of meditation.

On this day many years ago, I was training a client at his home, more specifically his garage. He had an impressive free weight setup with just about every machine and device that a well equipped gym would have. In addition, he had an enormous number of Olympic plates and dumbbells at his disposal and was a very dedicated lifter to boot. His garage was a large block building with no central heat. The only heat source was a space heater that used kerosene as a fuel source. Like most of my clients, this guy was a wonderful person, easy to get along with, and we developed a great rapport.

A normal exercise session should last about an hour. My client was a big man, around 6' 5" weighed around 290 lbs and lifted enormous weights. This guy was a great storyteller, and I knew I would be there at least 2 hours (an hour to lift and an hour to trade stories, one of the great rewards of my business). This was a very cold February day in Pennsylvania where the temperature with wind chill was 20 degrees below zero and the winds were howling outside. Well, as any good trainer would suggest, I wanted the place to be toasty warm, so he would not injure himself lifting. He fired up the space heater and sealed all the doors. There were no windows in his garage and I must say he did an excellent job of sealing the garage from drafts and air movement.

As the first hour went on, and the chemical fumes began to build in the garage, I felt myself start to wheeze. As I mentioned, he was a large man who had the structure to lift large amounts of weight. As part of my service, I always change the plates around for my clients and of course handed them the weight to lift.

As I began to ingest the fumes from the kerosene heater and lift hundreds and hundreds of pounds of weights repeatedly in this sealed area, the fumes entered my lungs and I felt them burn. Then my whole chest began to constrict and tighten. My throat started to close, and I could not get my air. I was going into a full blown asthma attack without my respirator to help me. My pride would not let me tell this guy, "hey I'm having an asthma attack, I need to cut your training session short and run to the hospital." I endured. I used my breathing techniques the best I could to control myself, but I needed to get help quickly because I could feel myself slipping.

Finally, the session was over, and by the time I collected my money and was back in my truck, I was in a full attack. When you are in full attack as I call it, your thinking process starts to shut down; decision-making is impaired and panic begins to envelop you. I tell people it is like drowning under water on dry land. At this point, I was undecided where to go: home, where I had my medication as well as comfort, or to the hospital in Pittsburgh. I was closer to home and decided to go for it. I started to drive home and I instinctively knew I was really close to a heart attack. I could feel my heart pounding in my chest as it tried to push through what little oxygen it could get. My body was oxygen deprived. I looked in the rear view mirror and saw that my lips were blue. I looked at my hands and my fingernails were blue. I knew I had to get some help soon, but I had a 25-minute drive ahead of me before I was home. I knew time was everything, and I needed to continue driving to get to my medication. I have been doing meditation so long that I can do it with my eyes open. This is a good thing if you are driving! First, I began to pray. I did not want to become a danger on the road. Thank God, there was no one else on the road at this time of day. I decided to slow down regardless if someone came up behind me. I did not have a car phone with me to call for help, besides what could I say? I prayed, Lord please allow me to make it home. I thought of my parents and of never seeing them again. I thought of my then girlfriend. I began to think, when I die will I be remembered at all and what will I be remembered for? Did I do good on Earth, did I help my fellow man or did I take advantage? Crazy thoughts. What is my purpose? Why am I here? If I survive, what will I do differently? I was not afraid to die. I had died before. Nevertheless, I instinctively knew that I was not finished with my purpose here on Earth yet. It was at this point when I did one of the healing meditations I discuss later, the White Tiger Meditation. This meditation has saved me numerous times from asthma attacks.

Healing Meditations Preparation

To begin, you must have at least tried to do the visualization and deep breathing methods before a crises hits. This is imperative to your progress at this level of belief and understanding. These are your ABCs to control your body to make the following meditations real and alive. If you do not have someone to read the meditation to you, you may want to record it, and play it for yourself until you have the sections committed to memory.

You can do this meditation sitting or standing. The most important thing is to relax and allow your musculature to relax. The only preparation to doing the following meditation is the following.

First, close the lower energy gate of your body so that energy no longer can flow out, but is trapped and stored. This area is called the perineum or CV-1 in Chinese Medicine. It is located between the genitalia and the anus. Closing this area is like squeezing the muscles for the Kegal exercises.

Second, place the tongue gently against the upper palate, next to the front teeth. This connects the two circuits of the human body like a positive and negative ends of a battery connected by copper. Notice this the next time you place batteries in your favorite toy or appliance. Now begin to relax, close your eyes and listen.

The Four Fundamentals

Use the following four visualization steps to relax and prepare for the healing meditation.

Air Passages: The Mind

One is Sun. Relax and imagine that you are on the beach. Hear the pounding of the surf and the smell of the salt air. Hear the gulls gently crying in the background against the surf. Look up into the sky and see the sun shining brightly down on the water. Now begin to feel the sun shine with its healing, rejuvenating warmth on the front of your face. Feel the warmth relaxing the tension in the facial muscles as the rays pour forth onto your skin and penetrate into the muscles, tendons and ligaments of your body. Relax your eyes, your cheeks, any tension in your jaw and your neck. The rays of sunlight are moving down your body to your chest and shoulders. Feel your body just hanging on the frame of your bones like a coat on a coat hanger. Now feel the life-giving warmth on your stomach, it penetrates deep into the tissues of the organs and with its touch heals any problems you may have. Now move the beam of light energy to your pelvis and relax the muscles from tension. Feel the area become warm and bathed with healing, penetrating heat from the sun. Move the healing beam of sunlight to the front of your thighs, your knees and finally to your shins and feet.

Feel the sun rays striking the back of your body, enveloping the back of your head. Feel the heat and the life-giving warmth flow down the shoulders, blissful warmth on the shoulder blades and the thick part of your back. Now relax and open up the back and the spine; feel the space between your ribs as you breath. Feel the deep heat penetrate into the very essence of your back and chest, lengthening and opening the tissues, uncurling any knots you might have and gradually giving yourself permission to allow the whole lower back to open up. Feel the spaces between your vertebra open and release any pinched or painful nerves; bathe them in healing heat. Now move your attention from the small of the back, down to the buttocks. Imagine healing, penetrating heat releasing all tightness, tension and pain. Feel the heat moving inward, down the back of your legs, your calves and into your heels.

Now feel the Sun directly over your head entering the very top of your skull and begin to warm and bathe the inside of your head with its life-giving energy. Feel the rays of light begin to pour down behind your eyes, enter your sinuses, and begin to open the throat. Remember, everything that the warming sunlight touches, it heals and relaxes back to a healthy, vibrant state. Allow the energy to descend into the lungs and heat the area so that you now begin to feel warmth inside your chest. Allow the sun's rays to further drop into your stomach, your small intestine and your colon. Feel the light, now split into two rays of equal proportions begin to filter down into the very bones of your pelvis and into the top of each thigh. Allow the pure energy to trace down the thighs to the knees, where it bathes the entire knee joint with warmth and soothing energy. Feel the ray enter your calves and move to the bottom of your feet, where it exits from the balls of your feet and forces itself back into the very Earth.

Two is Glue. The rays of the sun now are permeating the front of your entire body, your back, even the internal organs, and the very bone marrow itself. Feel the warmth, and a slight vibration begin to trickle from the sky above you permeating your body through the top of the head. Feel the connection you established between Heaven and Earth by opening up the bottom of the feet for the Sun's rays to escape. Pretend that your entire body is now an open river channel of light, flowing from top to bottom funneling the heat, warmth, and light from the sun to the bottom of your feet. Now, feel the bottom of your feet connect to the earth as the beam of light coming from the bottom of your feet pushes into the Earth, like a tree growing it's roots. Push the roots and tubulars deeper into the earth with each breath. Spread out the tubulars wider than you are tall and twice your height deep. You are now "glued" to the earth by your root system. You are connected between Heaven and Earth. Feel the energy pathway originating from the sky, moving through your body like a conduit, and entering the earth through your root system.

Three Is Free. Allow your body to now freely run pure white light energy from the heavens, through your body, and out through your feet like a stream of clean water washing all impurities with it. Cleanse your body from all infection, mucous, all pain, all the plaque within the artery walls, all the toxins that make you ill. Now feel the stream of clean water begin to warm itself by becoming part of your blood flow. Feel the blood cleansing itself of all impurities, all excess fat. Feel all the impurities and pain washing out through the bottom of your feet into the Earth through your roots. The earth will recycle all this negative energy and purify it. Feel the fresh clean oxygen permeating your very cells and nourishing them back to health. Be free from all that ails you.

Four Is Pore. Now that your body is free from all impurities and pain, recharge the body like a giant battery with pure clean energy. With each inhalation of the body, bring in all that is pure from nature. One of the miracles of nature is its ability to thrive and adapt to absolute chaos. To spawn new life where there was absolute destruction. Fire, flood, or volcanic action can NOT stop nature from re-growing, from surviving, from starting life anew. The power of living things to grow and multiply and to regenerate themselves is a special gift. You now have this ability. You can now pull into your body through your very pores the exact same vital energy that allows nature to regenerate itself. This life-giving energy permeates your skin through your pores, bathes your muscles, tendon and ligaments, revitalizes your blood and your spinal fluid, bathes your mind with hope and sinks deeply into the cavity of the body to revitalize your internal organs.

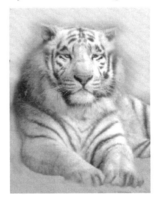

White Tiger Meditation

"Wisdom is the ability to denounce negative thought and patterns"

My martial arts instructor taught me this meditation when I was very young. I have used this meditation in many ways: through many asthma attacks and through stressful times in my personal and business life. It is one of the best meditations I know for when we are intimidated, frightened, overwhelmed and just plain scared of the unknown.

The white tiger is a rare and beautiful animal. Throughout history in Asia, the white tiger has had an air of mystery and magic associated with it. It has always symbolized courage and protection for those who respected its power.

Before you start, please take a moment to look at and memorize the white tiger picture. This picture is the white tiger I always envisioned. If this does not fit your perception, that's fine, but make sure your mind has a clear picture of the tiger that you want to be present in your meditation before you start. Allow yourself to be comfortable by either standing or by sitting in a comfortable chair. Allow your mind to settle for a moment by using the preparation techniques, and breathing techniques. Prepare a recording of the following, or have it read to you:

Picture yourself standing somewhere that you feel safe. This can be anywhere, in any place, in any time in your life. Feel the security of being safe and comfortable overwhelm you and start to override your fears and your doubts. Nothing can harm you here. Nothing can hurt you or cause you any pain. This is a sanctuary. Feel the security of love surround you. The warmth and the glow that being loved can bring to you. The feeling of when your mother hugged you as a child, or when your father held your hand as you walked across a busy street. Feel the power that this brings to you. Feel the importance of being connected to someone who cares about you.

This is your core line of defense against all that threatens, intimidates and bothers you.

Now look out to the horizon where the real world lies. You can't see the real world yet, but you know that it is out there, waiting for you. Out of the mist in a distance, you begin to see the shape of something moving. Upon looking closer, you see that it is a white tiger moving through blue mist. See the tiger moving toward you. You know instinctively, that this tiger is your friend, your protector. She is like the parents you knew would always be there for you, whenever you needed them. Examine the tiger and notice the size of her body. Her physical presence alone can frighten away anyone who would harm you. See the powerful muscles moving underneath her coat; observe her back and the powerful neck that makes this tiger one of the most revered and respected animals in the land. Notice the large paws walking silently and gracefully towards you. See the eyes, considered fierce by anyone who looks into them, except you. To you, she is a friend, a companion, a guardian. See the light reflect off the enormous white fangs and teeth projecting out of the large powerful jaws and neck. Now see that she, this magnificent white tiger protector, is a few feet away from you, and she begins to circle you. You trust the tiger implicitly with your life. She has her head turned toward the horizon to fend off anything that would trouble or worry you. You know that she will protect you, as she would protect her cub. She continues to circle you, to guard you. You begin to look to the horizon as the blue mist begins to drift away revealing outlines of the real world; the world that used to frighten you.

You notice that a second white tiger has started to circle you. This tiger has the same love for you as the first, only it is larger. Now both tigers circle you, their large heads and teeth facing the outside world. They will allow nothing ever to harm you. Listen and you can hear low rumbling in their throats. They are sending out an audible warning to anyone who comes near. Nothing can penetrate their shield. No power can overcome their protection and devotion to you. Look again to the horizon. See the world begin to take on more and more detail. See color and definition begin to appear. This scene can be whatever frightens you: work, getting up in front of an audience, taking that important test or interviewing for the big job. The white tiger stands for courage. With the tigers surrounding you, you have courage to do anything, to face your greatest fears, to become like the tigers themselves.

Now bring your attention back to the two tigers circling you. Notice that a third loyal white tiger has joined them and is circling you in the same direction as the other two. All of them are baring their teeth to anyone who would come near to harm you. See their claws ready to defend you in a moment's notice. Feel their combined power and protection. Feel the tiger's acceptance of who you are, and the good you stand for. Know that the three tigers are invincible, that they can overcome anything together with you. Know that they pledge their lives to you and will always guard you, circle you and protect you in every world. One tiger represents your physical body. The second tiger represents your emotional self, and the third tiger represents your spiritual nature.

Now the tigers begin to move around you faster and faster. They are now running full speed in a perfect circle around you, allowing nothing to penetrate their perimeter. All three tigers are moving so quickly now that they become a white blur surrounding you like a funnel cloud of protection. This cloud begins to move upward over your head and reaches a point 3 feet above you. You can no longer make out the bodies of the tigers as they have fused together into one huge vortex of power. The vortex is a bright white glow of energy that surrounds you like a teepee, from your feet to the top of your head. The energy begins to radiate up from your feet to the top of the teepee and begins to pour down into the top of your head, like pouring milk into a funnel. You now start to feel the courage of the three tigers permeate your mind, your thoughts and your body. All the attributes the tigers represents - courage, power, strength, and protection, on all three levels of body, emotion and spirit - now become yours as well. You are now the three tigers in spirit. They have fused with you to become part of you. They now become part of your personality, your attributes, your defense against the world.

At any given time, within a moment's notice the tigers can pour out from the top of your head and form a protective barrier to the rest of the world. They can never leave you because they are a part of you, as you are a part of them.

Crashing Wave Meditation

You can be seated or standing for this meditation, although I prefer to be standing. Close your eyes and relax.

Focus your attention on the front of your body and feel warm water run down over your face like a warm shower on a cold day, down your chest over your stomach, down the front of your legs to your feet. Feel the warm, healing water run down the back of your head, over the nape of your neck, over the top of your back. It relaxes each muscle group that it touches. Feel the water continue down the small of your back, healing any ache or pain you might have. Feel it continue down to the back of your legs, releasing the tension from your day. Feel the warm water circle your calves and flow down to the heels of your feet. Your body feels rejuvenated .

Begin to picture yourself at the beach on the ocean. Hear the waves crashing into the sand. Smell the salt air as the ocean ionizes the water into a fine mist. Allow the sounds of the sea gulls to fill the background of the pounding surf. Hear the rhythm of the ocean as the waves start sounding their path slowly out to sea. Within seconds, the surf is building and energizing the water into a deafening roar as the waves begin to rise high on the horizon and begin to curl under. As the sound increases, see the white foam begin to curl at the top. See the wave begin to crash down into the ocean as it roars toward the beach and laps at the sand you are standing on.

Air Passages: The Mind

Hear the rhythms and feel the vibration of Mother Nature's sounds. There is a certain predictable flow to the surf. Listen for it now and allow your body to relax in its consistency. Now in your mind, turn your back toward the surf. Still hear and feel the crashing of the surf in its continuous rhythm. Hear the waves starting way out at sea and begin to imagine that you are a rock standing freely in the water. Feel the warm sun-heated water rushing up your back slowly at first and then begin to increase in force. Feel the water crest at the top of your head and just like an ocean wave begin to curl over your forehead and fall down towards your feet in the sand. Now your breathing follows the same rhythmic pattern of the ocean. As the wave begins its ascent up your back, you will inhale deeply into the lower Dan tian, the energy area about three inches below the belly button. Feel your back expand and the oxygen to enter your lung sacs as they fill up with life-giving oxygen.

As each wave laps over your forehead, begin to exhale all the toxins and impurities from your body. Feel the water absorb all the worries and cares from your mind and begin to wash them away. Feel the mind relax, feel it clean off all the mud and sludge of worry. Feel the mud and sludge washing away with the ebbing wave out to sea, much like the sediment is pulled back away from the beach at the seashore. Continue to regulate your breath in this fashion until there are no more impurities being washed out to sea and only clean sparkling water is pouring down the front of your body. Inhale again, and feel the wave begin to caress the back of your legs, your lower back, your upper back and then up and over the top of your head.

The wave now begins to crash downward, but it is clean water with no debris in it. Remember that salt water is healing to the touch, and everything that this pure ocean water touches, begins to heal. Feel this pure water and earth energy now begin to enter into the core of your body, nourishing all your internal organs, bathing them with health and vitality. Feel the water now begin to settle in your lower Dan tian, and pool there much like a waterfall into a tropical pool of water. Feel this energy build in your lower Dan tian and energize the area.

Look into the distance, and see the sun reflecting off the ocean. See how the water almost takes on a white, sparkling, frothy look. As you inhale, feel the white froth rise up the spine over the back of the head and pour down into the lower Dan tian again. Feel the power emanate from the white water. Feel your entire torso become energized with pure water and light from the Earth. Feel the energy begin to heal all your past wounds and problems with healing light and energy from the ocean.

You can stay in this ocean as long as you need to. As you learn to quiet your mind a little more each time, enjoy the feeling of just breathing deeply and slowly for several minutes. No need to rush. This is your meditation. As long as you are getting some desired effect from it, you are doing it right. My words are here to guide you, to coach and to help you. There is no right or wrong. Just breathe, relax and be yourself. Concentrate on your breath. Feel it come into your body and rejuvenate and restore it.

Lung Expansion Meditation

"The ancestor to every action is a thought"

-Wayne Dyer

Sit back in a chair with your back supported and your legs bent comfortably so that your knees are below your hips.

Relax and notice your breathing. Is your breathing deep or shallow? Is your chest moving or is your stomach? How about the lower back, is it moving with your stomach? Take inventory of your body right now and feel if there is any tension. Does anything hurt? Is anything sore? This is your time to heal and to decompress. You deserve this time to yourself. You have to take time to refresh and rejuvenate yourself. This is your birthright to do so. So permit yourself to become relaxed. Forget about everything that happened to you today. Forget about everything except yourself for the next couple of minutes. Give yourself this time to heal.

Now bring your attention to your feet. Rotate them in all directions allow them to stretch. Think only about your feet. As soon as your attention begins to break, move your thoughts up to your calves. Flex them and then relax them. Notice the difference between tension and relaxation. Now, concentrate only on the feeling of relaxation. Move your concentration up your legs to your thighs. Squeeze the thighs by flexing the muscles, then relax them. Concentrate on the feeling of relaxation. Picture the muscles relaxing like ropes that were stretched tight and then given slack. Feel your muscles like ropes that have slack in them. Move your attention up to your waist and back. We are going to spend some time here because this is where the root of tension sometimes begins.

Focus your mind on the muscles of the waist. Bring your attention to your lower back area. Feel the muscles in your lower back. Are you holding the muscles in a position that is uncomfortable or unnatural? Relax the tension in the lower back and feel the chair push into your back. Feel your spine stretch. Feel the vertebras elongate and stack one on top of each other like blocks. Now bring your attention around to the front of the stomach. Release the tension in your stomach and allow your lower muscles, and your Dan tian (about three fingers below your stomach) to relax. It is okay to allow your stomach out; you no longer have to hold it in position. Now bring your attention back to your breath. Feel the air come into your nose, move down your chest and settle into your lower Dan tian. As you exhale, pretend you are blowing up a balloon. Let the air out of your lungs slowly. Your body may not be used to breathing this way, so if you have to, allow yourself to take a normal breath if it helps you relax more.

Continue to breathe deeply into the lower stomach or Dan tian and blow up the balloon as you exhale for several minutes. Feel all tension escape your body.

Now, move your concentration up your back to your shoulders. Notice if they are tense, slumped or just tight. Bring your attention to the muscles of the shoulder and chest area. Are you holding your shoulders tight or back? Bring your shoulders up to your ears, rotate them back and allow them to drop down naturally. As you do this several times, notice the tension removed from your neck and shoulders. Feel the muscles elongate. Feel the knots unravel and lengthen. Your muscles become longer because of this. Feel blood moving through the area again; as if a dam has now broken. Feel the area bathed in fresh blood and lymph. Picture the fresh clean blood moving through the area, washing and cleansing the area of all toxins and debris. Feel the area become warm.

Move your attention up to your neck and head. Relax your jaw muscles. Feel the muscles around your eyes relax. Feel your forehead and scalp loosen. Now breathe and feel clean fresh air enter your body.

With each inhalation, feel your lungs take in pure clean air and push the air down the chest into the stomach, three fingers below the bellybutton. As you exhale, feel the lungs push out all toxins that have entered your body. All that remains in your entire body is clean, healing energy. Every breath brings in more clean, pure energy. Breathe this way and focus on your breathing, bring all your concentration to your breath. The breath is your key to healing. Become one with your breath.

Bring your mind's attention to your breath. Envision the air you breathe as clean, pure, healing, white mist. Picture this several times, breathing in the same deep controlled manner as you had before. See the air traveling through your body. Bring your attention to the passages of your nose, down the airway of your throat, down deep into your chest, deep inside the caverns and tunnels of your lungs. Now feel the bronchiole tubes open wider and wider each time you inhale. Allow them to expand and relax just as your body did in the beginning. You can control your breathing, making it deeper and deeper. You are in control of your body. You can control your heart rate, your blood pressure, and your ability to breathe evenly and deeply. You can allow your body to work more efficiently. Each time you inhale, you are training your body to breathe deeply and expand your lungs to a greater and greater volume. Feel the lungs working more efficiently, effortlessly, without any discomfort. Just relax and give your body time to adapt to this new feeling. Be patient with yourself. If your mind wanders away, try not to dwell on those thoughts, but gently guide it back to your breath. Return to visualizing your lungs opening and expanding the bronchiole tubes. Feel the lungs widen like huge pipes bringing in clean, healing energy that rushes into your body and envelopes every muscle, every tissue, every organ, every cell that comprises you. Every exhalation expels the pathogens you desperately want to get rid of.

Goals

How long should you meditate? As we discussed in the exercise portion of Chapter 7, you should gradually work up to your potential. In the first month the breathing/visualization will be difficult to do for even ten minutes. By the third month, you should be able to hold the visualization for at least twenty minutes. At the end of six months, optimistically, you will be able to hold the visu-

Air Passages: The Mind

alization/ breathing for 30 minutes. Again, it is not the goal to reach the time limit, but to reach the state of relaxation and rhythmic breathing. This is where the benefits lie. However, you should notice your concentration abilities increasing by the third or fourth month.

Meditation and visualization are fundamental tools for asthmatics, who, as I did in the story, may fall into unpredictable circumstances that precipitate an asthma attack. Without these tools, we are a time bomb waiting to explode into a full-blown asthma attack.

CHAPTER 11
Prednisone & Albuterol

Prednisone is a Godsend and is of the devil itself. Having been on prednisone most of my life, I can tell you that it produces a roller coaster ride of emotions, including relief and despair. The drug is miraculous in how it makes you feel after an episode of severe itching or rash, but coming off of it is a whole other matter. Staying on prednisone brings its own banquet of ills, and easing yourself off of its hold will test your mental stamina and patience like nothing else on this earth.

Prednisone relieves the pain for many people with arthritis, and for many young people who have bronchial asthma or allergies, skin conditions (poison ivy or oak), joint and muscle disorders and even certain kinds of cancer. Like all "miracle drugs," when it first came out in the '60s prednisone was very expensive, as much as $25 per prescription, but now is relatively inexpensive.

I used prednisone for my asthma and allergies, especially my skin allergies. My skin would become so inflamed and red that I looked like a lobster. The skin would actually break open and crack, bleed at the same time, and get infected. The only thing that helped was prednisone. This drug also helped to control my severe asthma symptoms. What a wonderful drug, I thought.

In the '60's, Prednisone was one of the greatest advances in drug therapy, in my opinion, for the asthma and allergy sufferer. At that time, there were no inhalator steroids to speak of. Prednisone was the drug of choice then, and in some cases still is today, because it works wonderfully. Many asthmatics now use inhaled steroids instead of prednisone, but it is still the physicians drug of choice for some patients.

Prednisone actually mimics the bodies' production of cortisol, a naturally occurring steroid manufactured by your adrenal glands, which sit on top of your kidneys. The adrenals do quite a few things including:

1. Regulating body salts to ensure the fine balance between sodium and potassium and fluid retention
2. Reducing inflammation in the lungs and elsewhere on the body
3. Helping the body metabolize carbohydrates, proteins and fats
4. Releasing added steroids as protection from physical stress
5. Helping to control heart rate and blood pressure

If you have been on prednisone, ask your doctor about every-other-day administration with twice the dosage. This has a benefit of not suppressing the pituitary and adrenal glands (a common problem); their suppression can cause Cushing's Disease, or stunted growth in children. Cushing's Disease is characterized by obesity, with most of the fat deposited around the midriff. Other common problems are bruising due to thinning skin, osteoporosis, high blood pressure, and electrolyte imbalances. Many physicians recommend taking prednisone early in the morning because the body manufactures its own natural version of prednisone drug during daylight hours and production gradually tapering off overnight.

If you have never looked up prednisone in the <u>Physicians Desk Reference</u>, or PDR, you might be shocked what you find. It comes under several names, such as Deltasone, Meticorten and Prednicen-M. Sterapred is prednisone in a tapering 21 or 12 day dosage and there is also a liquid form. Prednisone comes in 1, 2.5, 5, 10, 20, and 50 mg. tablets that are gluten-free. If you are allergic to gluten (the insoluble protein of most grains which makes flour rise) you may want to watch for it in other medications. Prednisone is used for so many things that there probably is a book out there that is just on prednisone. Besides asthma and allergies, it is also used for: bursitis, arthritis, psoriasis, dermatitis, rhinitis, leukemia, ulcerative colitis, and acute multiple sclerosis. My good friend Dr. Fraley used to call it a "miracle drug," because it seems to be good for just about everything that ails you.

Then, there is prednisone's dark side. Short-term use of corticosteroid therapy is usually not a hazard to your health. Long-term use, however, can do pretty serious damage. How long is long term? That seems to vary depending on who you talk to. From my experience, after 2 weeks of prednisone you will start to see some changes, especially puffiness in the face and water retention. The first thing you will notice however, is the increase in appetite. It seems that you never want to stop eating and drinking. Between the water retention and puffiness, and the increase in appetite, no wonder most people on steroids have a weight problem, if not obesity. Last year I saw a little girl on television who was having a multi-organ transplant. The poor little thing had the classic "moon face" that occurs when a patient is on steroids. Weight gain and puffiness is bad enough, but what's going on behind the scenes is what always concerned me most.

SERIOUS SIDE EFFECTS / LONG TERM EFFECTS

Infections

Frequently asthma teams up with allergies that manifest on the skin. Prednisone still seems to be a favorite way of treating this condition. Prednisone's effect on the immune system is critical. It decreases your body's ability to fight infection and sets you up for increased susceptibility to acquire infection. Staph (staphylococcus) infection is one way that prednisone, Deltasone, and any other corticosteroid can creep up on you. Staph is located on our skin pretty much all the time, in our skin glands and in all the mucus that the body naturally creates. Since staph is already on our skin, it is one of the chief ways burn patients get infections. For sustained users of prednisone, staph can be just as troublesome. Dermatitis can result from low immune function and when coupled with staph can lead to a condition known as staphylodermatitis. Pimples will often erupt along with the dermatitis.

Chicken Pox

Getting infections or catching the common cold are unpleasant, but contracting chicken pox can be life-threatening for someone on long-term steroid use. When I contracted chicken pox, we were not sure at first what it was because I had had so many infections previously. By the time we got to the doctor a day or two later, the damage was complete. Prednisone seemed to make the chicken pox virus mutate into a super pox. My pox marks were the size of half-dollars. This can happen to adults and to children. Another evil culprit is measles. Measles also can have life-threatening complications for people on steroids and should be seen by a physician immediately.

Drying Out

Most of my life I have tried to be off corticosteroids, but unfortunately, I have only managed to be off them for a few years. The change in seasons, stress, and exposure to chemicals or allergens, all seem to exacerbate my allergy and asthma symptoms. Visiting someone who has a cat or whose house is filled with dusty rugs and knickknacks or someone cutting brush next to your house as well as other exposures can all build up and lead to an eruption symptoms. For someone who is immune system stressed, often minor irritations build up, and then the big one hits and sends you over the edge. This is universally true of many severe sufferers of allergies and asthma.

Steroids in general suppress your immune system making you susceptible to disease and infections from bacteria, viruses, parasitic, and fungus. Even short-term doses in the elderly can lead to bone density depletion such as osteoporosis. Steroids can also lead to water retention and muscle loss.

Make sure you tell your doctor if you have or in the past have had: AIDS, heart disease, high blood pressure, liver or kidney disease, diabetes, inflammation of throat, stomach, or intestines, glaucoma, fungal infections, myasthenia gravis, osteoporosis, herpes infection or tuberculosis.

Do not stop taking this drug suddenly; the dosage must be lowered gradually! Do not drink alcohol of any type while on this drug as it can lead to an ulcer. If you have any surgery or extensive dental work planned, make sure that the doctor knows you are on this drug. Do not take aspirin or Ecotrin while taking prednisone.

Call your doctor if you experience:

> Decreased or blurred vision
> Frequent urination
> Hallucinations
> Increased thirst
> Depression or mood swings
> Skin rash or hives

After long term use:

> Persistent abdominal pain
> Acne or other skin problems
> Bloody or black tarry stool
> Rounding of the face
> Increased blood pressure
> Swelling of feet or legs
> Weight gain
> Irregular heartbeat
> Muscle cramps or pain
> Unusual tiredness or weakness
> Pain in back, ribs, arms or legs
> Muscle weakness
> Nausea or vomiting
> Thin shiny skin
> Unusual bruising
> Wounds that will not heal

After you stop taking the drug, call your doctor immediately if you have:

> Abdominal or back pain
> Dizziness or fainting
> Low fever
> Persistent loss of appetite
> Muscle or joint pain
> Nausea or vomiting
> Shortness of breath
> Unexplained headaches
> Unusual tiredness or weakness
> Unusual weight loss
> Depression

Indigestion
Increased appetite
Trouble sleeping
Flushed face
Nosebleeds
Increase in facial or body hair

While you are on this drug, it is a good idea to have periodic tests to measure blood or urine glucose concentration, and blood levels of potassium, sodium and calcium. You should also have stool tests for blood loss, and hypothalamus and pituitary secretion test as well as eye examinations.

Some individuals may end up crying at the simplest frustration, or become so over-sensitive that nothing anyone says is the right thing. Others may have severe depression and even self-destructive thoughts. The <u>Physician's Desk Reference</u> states that "Psychic derangement" may appear when corticosteroids are used, ranging from euphoria, insomnia, mood swings, personality changes, and severe depression, to psychotic manifestations. Also, existing emotional instability or psychotic tendencies may be aggravated by corticosteroids. I have known a lot of people on prednisone and they all had the side effect of mood swings. Many times people are not even aware of their moods changing, but the people around them sure are. Prednisone or any corticosteroids are powerful drugs and their side effects are many. Please treat it with an enormous amount of respect.

Trying to get off long-term administration of prednisone takes all your mental and physical energy. Being on steroids is very difficult. It is imperative to wean yourself off gradually otherwise you will experience such physical withdrawal symptoms and emotional upset that your very well-being could be in jeopardy. Always work with your physician and your pharmacist when trying to wean yourself. I have found that certain times of the year and/or if you are under a lot of stress can affect a withdrawal schedule. Sometimes I would have to stay on a particular dose for weeks; otherwise, I would begin to have skin eruptions again. Communicate special circumstances to your physician; who should consider them. If not, you may want to look for another physician.

One of the most noticeable side effects of coming off prednisone is the nervousness that seems to overwhelm you. It feels like you are "right on your last nerve," and the simplest of things seem to upset and bother you. It is as if all the mature coping skills that you have acquired over the years have gone out the window. Patience is gone, the jitters inside are non-stop, and your temper is just waiting for an opportunity to vent on some poor unsuspecting victim of circumstance. My wife says that I am having a "PMS attack" when this happens. I just warn her ahead of time that I'm "getting off the pred," and she knows what to expect. Please explain this to the people who love and care about you and ask them to have a little extra patience with you and your short fuse. They may not realize that what's happening to you is a chemical adjustment/reaction and that it's not your fault.

Dealing with the public, especially if you are in a service-oriented business can be trying in your altered state. With all the different personality types that you come in contact with in a service-oriented business, the days can feel very long. You have to keep telling yourself, "It will all be over soon." Most importantly, try to get enough sleep at this time. Being tired and weaning yourself of drugs is a prescription for disaster. We all have different requirements for sleep. Some can feel great on six hours, others need eight to nine to feel human. Let experience be your guide.

Your appetite may change as well. Sometimes you will crave the very thing you are allergic to. Many comfort foods are known to be highly allergic. Chocolate, milk products, peanuts (think of the sundae you have been craving) are all foods known to be trouble for allergic people. Be careful of this, as you know yourself and your body better than anyone. Other times I have lost my appetite all together, or everything tastes bland and boring. This is when you eat to be functional rather than for pleasure. Try to eat at regular intervals; about every four to five hours is good. Eat smaller meals (snacks would be a better term for measurement) of good healthy food that you are not allergic to. See Chapter 5 on diet for more information. You do not want to stress the body any more by not providing fuel it needs to function properly.

I have found that a high protein, low-fat diet with minimal amount of carbohydrates is the best way to combat the inevitable weight gain. This may be partially true because the glucocorticoids promote the composition or buildup of carbohydrates from noncarbohydrate sources (protein). This makes for more glucose or blood sugar available for the body (muscles) to use. However if too much blood sugar is available, then stress begins to mount on the pancreas which produces insulin.[2] Insulin is the hormone that carries the blood sugar into the muscle cells and liver and also promotes the storage of fat. Therefore, since the body is already converting protein to glucose via amino acids (the building blocks of protein used for repair of the body) why over saturate the body with more carbohydrates (glucose) which places more strain on the pancreas.

A good multivitamin is imperative at this time. The mineral's potassium, calcium, and magnesium are especially important because prednisone depletes them from the body. The body also begins to store salt and water (bloating), which is why exercise is so important as a natural means to sweat out extra salt and water.

Martial arts are a saving grace for me at this time, my practice gives me the mental discipline and reserve to combat all the ills that prednisone so indiscriminately bestows. Use your exercise program to help you in this manner.

Water is especially crucial for weaning off the corticosteroids. When you start to come off the drug, as well as after you have taken the drug awhile, you will notice how dry and flaky your skin becomes. If you have dry skin to begin with, and you are on prednisone, you should buy stock in all cream and moisturizing companies. Keep a bottle of water at your desk at work and carry one with you in your briefcase or purse. Take the opportunity to sip water throughout the day, and at night keep some at your bedside. I mentioned previously that I drink coffee for my asthma control. If you are a coffee drinker, since coffee is a diuretic, drink two mugs of water for every mug of coffee, this will make sure your body is hydrated enough.

The only successful way I have ever weaned myself off steroids for a long period of time (defined as a year or more) is through the use of an herbal tincture that I created (see Chapter 6 on antioxidants and my herbal tincture) and the use of Qigong breathing therapies (upcoming chapters). I have tried and used everything (with and without physician's approval) that you can possibly imagine and more, but these are the only two modalities that have worked for me.

When I tell western physicians how many years I was on prednisone, they look in disbelief. They know that by this time it should have killed me or left me physically deformed. It is the things that I write about in this book that has made all the difference between dying and living with a good quality of life.

Albuterol

For the last 20 years, most asthmatics have carried with them a drug called Albuterol that is a lifesaver. Several other aliases of Albuterol are Ventolin, Proventil, Salbutamol, or Volmax. The portable aerosol canister that allows you to self-administer a drug that relaxes the bronchial tubes is an amazing testament to the miracles of modern science. No doubt, it has saved many, many lives and the people responsible for its invention should be credited.

However, like everything else, Albuterol also has its downfalls as well. Some of the known side effects are tremors, nausea, headache, epistaxis, increased heart rate, increased blood pressure, dizziness, nervousness, and vomiting. Cases of urticaria, rash, bronchospasm, hoarseness, throat swelling and sleeplessness all have been reported with the use of Albuterol, so it is not the panacea that everyone thinks it is.

The most important point about Albuterol is this: prolonged use and frequent use will increase your heart rate and blood pressure… fact. So, what are our options? Well, asthma itself is not going away, I would never want anyone to be without an inhaler for emergencies. The fact is most people will use their inhaler more frequently as they get older so we have an inevitable increase in heart rate and blood pressure. People are then medicated for that. How do we interrupt this vicious cycle?

We must learn to override our autonomic nervous system and take control back by using meditation. If we do not learn to control our internal pharmacy, then we are at risk of being dictated to by the external pharmacy of inhalators and corticosteroids. Notice, I am not saying throw away the rescue medication, but I am reminding you that if you continue to/or must use this drug, then at least take precautions for your long term health.

The new kid on the block is a new inhalator called Xopenex. The same side effects of nervousness, tremors, headaches, dizziness, and heart palpitations have been reported with additional side effects of leg cramps and chest pain.

Air Passages: Prednisone & Albuterol

These new and old drugs are wonderful, but not without a price. Invest in yourself. The bottom line is this: Keep your rescue medications handy at all times, but do something proactive rather than just relying on the medication to do it all for you. Asthmatics need to adhere to diet control, stress management, purgation and meditation as part of their ongoing lifestyle.

The next several chapters will outline a form of medicine that, in my opinion, rivals and sometimes exceeds western medicine.

1) American Medical Association Essential Guide to Asthma; page 148
2) Biology, Second Edition chapter 41; page 923

CHAPTER 12

Chinese Medicine as Therapy

This section deals primarily with Chinese Medicine as I have learned it from many different teachers. There are two treatment methods that I have found useful in the Chinese medical system for asthma and allergy control. First, is the Chinese system of Qigong and second, is herbal medicine. I do know that many people have used acupuncture for the treatment of asthma with great success. I have also tried acupuncture, but it was not effective for me. It truly depends on how advanced your asthma/allergies are and perhaps the level of education of the acupuncturist. I will devote separate chapters to Qigong, specifically Medical Qigong and herbal medicines. Actually, both herbal remedies and Qigong need to be exployed together for optimal results in severe asthma and allergy treatment.

To be clear on my intent here, I must first say that Western doctors are the front line in asthma defense for acute attacks and emergency medicine. If I am going into anaphylactic shock, I want to be transported by ambulance to an ER or have a shot of epinephrine to save my life. The Eastern methods, however, use a vastly different approach, grounded in the belief that the cycle of allergy and asthma can even be reversed out of the body and in some cases cured. In other words, if you are having an asthma attack and you turn blue in the lips, get to the hospital. However, if you want to work on reducing your symptoms incrementally over time, so that each attack of asthma and allergies is progressively less and less, seek a Chinese Medical Doctor (OMD) or specifically a Doctor of Medical Qigong (DMQ).

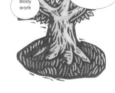

Four Branches of Chinese Medicine

In the following pages, I will be talking about one of the most profound and effective healing systems that has ever been recorded in the history of humankind. The system of Chinese Medicine (CM) with its four branches combines the intellectual and spiritual wealth of empirical knowledge spanning a minimum of five thousand years. This empirical knowledge was gained through trial and error, human provings, and demonstrated action and reaction. And from it evolved the planet Earth's first written and documented medical system, a system that is still in use today.

An Appointment with a Chinese Doctor

If you make an appointment with a practitioner of Chinese Medicine, certain terminology will be used that might sound confusing in that you will recognize the words used, but they will be referencing concepts that don't seem to make sense to you.

When Western medicine uses the word lungs, for example it generally means the organ. In Chinese Medicine, "Lungs" is an entire system. I will capitalize the Chinese names for Lungs as well as other Chinese medical names. I will explain how Chinese Medicine understands asthma in the context of the Five Yin Organs, but don't diagnose yourself. Consult a trained professional practitioner of acupuncture, herbals or Medical Qigong.

Chinese medicine does not diagnose a disease as western medicine does. It looks for the imbalances of the body and adjusts them to achieve an harmonious interplay. This imbalance is the foundation of Chinese disease-pattern-identification. Chinese Medicine uses many tools to locate and understand imbalance: the nine basic pulses, tongue diagnosis, face and eye diagnosis, five element theory, and, most importantly, intently listening to and watching the patient.

For extrinsic asthma, there usually are four different general diagnoses in Chinese Medicine: Heat, Cold, Phlegm, and Wind. If there is deficiency involved, as there usually is with asthma and allergies that start at a young age, the organs affected are usually Lung, Kidneys, and Spleen. In addition, Chinese diagnoses will take into account different kinds of mucous including, thick, thin, yellow or clear.

Long before the ancient Egyptians were building the great pyramids, the ancient Chinese were already obsessed with medicine. Through the various sects of Taoism comes to us oral, and in many cases, written traditions that have been carefully handed down with great dedication and precision. Their healing systems have endured the ultimate test of time and have kept the world's largest population healthy for thousands of years.

Air Passages: Chinese Medicine as Therapy

The classical medical texts of the "Nan-ching," written in the first century A.D. and their predecessors, "Huang-ti nei-ching su wen" and "Huang-ti nei-ching ling-shu," are still studied today by doctors of Chinese medicine (even M.D.'s) for insight into modern medical problems such as biological warfare and AIDS.

With such a history of success, it amazes me that more of the 18 million sufferers of asthma in the United States, are not utilizing classic Chinese Medicine seriously for insight into their allergies and asthma and its maintenance. Moreover, in this day of instant information, why aren't western physicians explaining these vital and life saving techniques (specifically Medical Qigong) to the masses in clear terms?

You may have noticed that I refer to Chinese Medicine and not Traditional Chinese Medicine (TCM), and I will try to elaborate on the differences between the systems. The Chinese Medicine that I am referring to is not necessarily the same as what is taught in TCM colleges in the United States, Europe or Australia for that matter. "Traditional Chinese Medicine" is relatively new conglomerate of various concepts and practices that Mao Se Tsueng thought would be a viable means of selling the indigenous Chinese Medical System of Healthcare to the West in a nice, neat package. Actually, many of the medical systems that grew out of the vastly different provinces of China were eliminated with this merger. In my studies with many physicians of Chinese medicine, I have noticed that much of what is taught in the United States is not the complete system, but an abbreviated one. For example, acupuncture has been gaining popularity over the last several years in North America but, unfortunately for us, it is not as powerful as it could be if it were taught here with all of its original teachings intact. For those of you practicing acupuncture, what I am referring to for example, is using the Divergent meridians as a complete treatment system like the twelve primary channels, or using the Luo channels as means to treat psychoemotinal disorders.

One method of teaching did survive the medical book burning and the enormous uncalculated loss of knowledge from the Cultural Revolution in China. That means of survival is the oral traditions kept alive by the Taoists priests. Here the complete teachings are intact because they were never written down in the first place. These priests were taught and trained from the time they were toddlers. Some were taught by family members, others were adopted into families of priests who were also versed in medicine. The teachings were passed down this way for generations. One of my most revered teachers is an eighty-eighth generation Taoist priest whose accumulation of medical knowledge, both east and west, seems immeasurable. Qigong and, especially, Medical Qigong, is a system of self-healthcare that has been preserved in these oral traditions.

Chinese Medicine involves the balance of nature internally within our body as well as our body balanced with nature externally. Some refer to this as the microcosmic balance within the macrocosmic balance. This interplay between body and nature involves our physical microcosm, our emotional microcosm, and our spiritual microcosm. For someone with allergies, asthma or immune dysfunction, this balance becomes an important concept for successfull regulation of our health, and even our survival.

In the Beginning.....

Understanding Chinese Medicine becomes an adventure unto itself. Because we are not raised with its ways of thinking or its vocabulary, its study can at first be difficult; it can make your brain "hurt". Other times its pragmatic and simple explanations for something very difficult can be so refreshing in today's high tech information-packed world, that you start to wonder why you were never educated in this fashion before.

In order for this book to work as a teaching guide for you, you will need to familiarize yourself with some basic concepts found in Chinese Medicine as well as thoughts utilized by many indigenous cultures around the world today. Bear with me as we go through some new terminology that will seem very foreign to you. The same would be true if you were to begin the study of computers, for example, but had never had any exposure before.

Let's pose the question of "where did everything start from?" to a room full of lay people from around the world and include scientists of physics, quantum physics, biology and astronomy as well as teachers of every faith and religion known on the planet. What do you think would happen in that room? I am not a betting man, but I would lay all my money on the fact that many people in that room would be in disagreement with each other! I would also bet the "discussion" would grow more heated as our cross section of experts began to debate more passionately.

The Chinese concept of Wuji (translated as absolute nothingness) does not attempt to explain how everything started, but just accepts that this is just so. The Chinese use the term Wuji to refer to a state of nothingness, of pure openness, or void, or emptiness where no boundaries exist. Other terms people use to try to relate to Wuji include: the nameless, the great mother, the one, the source. Some refer to this as God. What is unique about the concept of Wuji is that the Chinese believe that you can return to it in every waking hour of your life and experience it, but you can't describe it because it is beyond description of words and articulated thought. A very famous Chinese philosopher named Lao Tzu once said, "That which can be named is not the eternal name" and "The nameless is the mother of Heaven and Earth." Some things just have to be experienced in a humanistic sentient way, if only for a few minutes, but a person can still write or think about them for a lifetime. This is Wuji. Don't worry, Chinese medicine does get easier!

Qi

Well, maybe after this next concept is over with, then it will get easier. Of all the new concepts that Chinese Medicine has introduced us to, none is greater than the concept of Qi. Qi means "life energy." Qi, Chi, or Ki (pronounced Chee) is spelled many different ways with the same meaning. What is Qi? That is a very difficult question to answer because this is an Asian term for which there is no direct translation in English. As with many Chinese to American translations, this is loosely defined, as there is no parallel word in English for "Qi." Let us analyze a little deeper this concept of Qi.

The first Chinese book detailing chi or Qi is the "I Ching" (Book of Changes 1122 B. C.). Qi can be described as the life force that permeates every living entity. In many ancient cultures there is a universal belief that the Earth itself is a living entity. Think of "Mother Earth" in Native American and Inuit cultures. My intent here is not to prove or disprove this line of thinking, but to state that this logic has been in existence since the evolution of man, and continues to this day.

Qi roughly means the vapor, breath, and energy. In Taoism, Qi is the life force or the spirit that pervades and pulses through all living things. It is this primordial energy that sustains us, brings us great health and well-being or its weakening or loss brings sickness and death. Therefore the strength or the vitality of one's Qi can be measured by the quality of life one has.

There is a saying in Chinese Medicine: There will be no pain or disease if the Qi flows smoothly and evenly. There are two basic types of Qi: Yin Qi and Yang Qi. These two types must be balanced in the body, one cannot overpower the other. Chinese thought is almost a common sense approach to health care, in that more does not necessarily mean better, nor does abstinence. It is interesting to note that the Chinese do not believe in prolonged fasting (days), nor do they believe in overeating, as both they believe will injure the Qi. Makes sense to me.

Understanding of Qi, I predict, will one day be acknowledged as a great breakthrough of science; much like the more recent discovery of immune system identification. Before the immune system was defined as a functional unit at all, doctors believed that various organs associated with the immune system were "useless." The thymus gland, spleen, adenoids and appendix were all considered "extra" parts left over from a period when primitive man needed them. Well, we still need them, just as we need Qi.

Meridians

The meridians or pathways are areas of consistant, higher concentrations of Qi, rather than all or nothing idea. Qi permeates the entire body through a network of channels (meridians) that are the primary transporter of Qi from the body's surface to the very internal organs and back again. The meridians are more of a flow pattern/process than an actual physical structure. We are speaking of the subtle energy of the body. In other words, Qi is everywhere in the body; however, certain areas have a higher concentration or lower concentration. Along these higher concentration pathways are "points" where we apply pressure or needle these points as in acupuncture, we can affect the entire pathway of energy and thereby the whole body.

Recently Dr. Helene Langevin from the University of Vermont may have found the reason why the meridian system used in Chinese Medicine, and specifically in acupuncture, may have escaped confirmation by western medical doctors. She notes in a paper published in The Anatomical Record, that acupuncture points have a tendency to correspond to where connective tissue is the thickest. Dr. Langevin states, "Connective tissue forms a web that runs continuously throughout the body." This connective tissue, long understood by bodyworkers, contains nerve endings that when stimulated in the right leg, may feel or affect the torso for example.

Since we have not developed instruments delicate enough to detect Qi in its purest sense, we usually speak of its by-products: heat, light, and electromagnetic energy. Perhaps if we break Qi down to Western concepts, we can better understand Qi, and thereby believe in the therapeutic benefits of its cultivation. New terminology from western science describese Qi as bioelectricity.

Using state-of-the-art imaging and newly developed computers, a new system of MRI scanning called Nuclear Magnetic Resonance Imaging (NMRI) measures the induced changes in magnetic polarity of the body cells, specifically the blood flow, blood volume and the relative oxygenation of the cells. Since Qi flows with the blood, this is a great beginning. Through this new technology we can see the effect of acupuncture and Qi manipulation on the limbic system or the emotional core of the human nervous system. The specific area of the brain affected is called the amygdala sometimes called the "seat of emotions." Manipulating the Qi through Qigong or acupuncture calms the emotions of fear, anger, sadness and pain, which in turn calms the amygdala. It is the amygdala, by signaling other parts of the brain through neurohormones, that causes the stress response and pain!

Simply and scientifically speaking, Qi is a bioelectromagnetic energy enveloping the body. Many people describe Qi as wavelike or in the form of light. Qi and matter maintain energy that may not yet have been unlocked. For example, when we burn natural gas in our homes for heating, the gas in its natural state does not give off heat, but when burned for fuel, it unlocks and gives off tremendous heat, enough to heat our house.

Isaac Newton's law of conservation of mass states that mass cannot be created or destroyed, although the matter contained within the mass can be transformed from one type to another. Like matter, Qi can never be destroyed, but just takes on different forms or is recycled, if you will. Qi is not something that is tangible but like the oxygen we breathe, we will definitely know something is wrong when there is a lack of it. So too, will you notice if your Qi becomes weak, blocked, depleted or out of balance. You will become sick, run down, your clarity of mind will diminish, and your body will begin to give you symptoms of disease that we can then begin to diagnose with Western methods. Understanding Qi is the basis of Chinese medicine.

When split, a simple atom releases an incredible amount of energy, yet, the atom is something we never see. In the human body, Qi is derived from the air, water and food that we ingest (postnatal Qi) plus the original Qi (Yuan Qi) given to us by our parents at conception (genetics). The energy within the food and air is broken down in our body through biochemical reactions and then given off as heat and/or bioelectromagnetic energy. Once produced this way, the unneeded excess energy is stored as fat by the body until energy, or calories, is needed. Calories in Western science are actually measured units of stored heat.

The two most common ways to feel Qi is through heat or light and sometimes both together. Heat is felt in the body by the resistance to the movement of Qi; an analogy is the working of an electric stove burner. In an electric stove, the electricity moves through the coils and the coils begin to heat up. It is not the Qi or electricity itself that causes the heat, but the movement through the object (your body or the coils) and the effect of resistance that cause heat. Many people who practice developing their Qi to a higher level (Qigong) first feel the heat in their hands.

The concept of Qi is next on the world's most difficult concepts list. Qi is what is born out of the Wuji, as the first primordial energy in what we currently call the Universe. Qi moves first, before there is any movement on any plane of existence whether that be an ocean wave about to crest, or a neutrino particle passing through the Earth's core, or the orbit of the planets in our solar system, Qi initiates movement. Incidentally, physicists are in awe of what these neutrinos are and what they can do. If you had a steel plate a million miles thick, a neutrino would pass right through it! The more modern physicists understand and experiment, theorize and postulate, the more the ancient Chinese concepts of Qi and energy are making sense to them. As we re-write the world of physics in the

21st century by understanding quantum theory and mechanics, the more we can scientifically believe in Qi.

Qi is what moves before we have a thought, an emotion, sensory input or an understanding of what you are reading here. All energies emanate from Qi, whether that is light, heat, magnetism, electricity, etc, and are then sustained by Qi. Lack of Qi will cause the degradation of the entity until enough Qi is lost that the Qi returns back to the source, causing the death of the entity. As the first law of physics states: "energy cannot be created or destroyed, it just changes forms."

Qi is what gives living creatures their life force and metabolism. Metabolism is sustained by strong Qi, weak Qi reduces metabolism. So you can start to see the implications of Qi and health from an energetic or even a physics standpoint. I have even used these concepts of Qi in weight loss programs that work profoundly. Each person manifests Qi in a unique way based on the 5-element theory and Yuan Qi. Therefore I can't give you a generic weight-loss program that will be effective. Weight loss from a Qi perspective must be coached individually.

YIN and YANG

So now that we have a concept of Qi, we have to understand how Qi manifests itself as it begins to move through different planes. Qi moves like water and flows, circles and surges, but as soon as it manifests itself, it divides into Yin and Yang qualities. Yin and Yang constitutes the classic dichotomy used in so many ways to describe the differences between man and women, night and the day, heaven and the Earth, and the inside of the body and the outside of the body.

Yin and Yang compliment each other. Neither is more powerful or better than the other, but together construct balance by their very existence. Yin and Yang create our polarity of definition. You only know if something is hot or cold by having something to compare it with, a relationship. Thus we know stillness by its lack of movement. We know night because we know day, or as soon as you have a front of an item defined you must then have a back - and visa versa. Understanding Yin and Yang becomes a model for putting things in perspective. Yin and Yang should transform evenly and flow in order for there to be harmony and homeostasis. If there is an abrupt change such as going from Yin to over-whelming Yang, then there will be a great deal of discomfort or even pain. Think of going from several hours in a pitch-black room (Yin) into extremely bright sunlight (Yang), and of how your vision and your eyes would react. A disruption of harmony can be seen in the disruption of the breathing patterns of asthma sufferers, the emotions (becoming overwhelmingly angry or frightened), and even in the body's re-action to fight, fright or flight and stress. All these are definitions and relationships of Yin to Yang.

The words Yin and Yang are sometimes used in our culture, but few westerners understand their use in a medical context. Many people link Yin with the female or darkness and Yang with the male and light. The top of the body is considered Yang and the lower Yin. The back is Yang and the front is Yin. If the body is too Yang, then the Yin aspects will be weak. An entire college class could be devoted to Yin and Yang in medical diagnosis, but it is neccessary to remember individual symptoms are secondary to the understanding of the person as a whole.

Unlike Western medicine, there are no structural dichotomies in Chinese medicine. The Chinese are concerned with processes and influences rather than structure and exact orientation. Yin and Yang are concepts more than they are actual substances.

Most people in the West think of Yin and Yang as opposites, which is true, but like so many eastern concepts, that is only part of the story. Think of the familiar Yin and Yang symbol in which black resides in white and white within black. Black and white complement each other and are codependent. Yin and Yang are about relationship. Yin and Yang can be used to define the relationship one part of the body has to another, the relationship the body has to the mind, or even more intangibly, the relationship the spirit has with

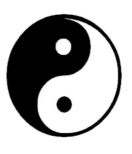

Yin	**Yang**
Water	Fire
Wet	Dry
Dark	Light
Stillness	Activity
Inside	Outside
Front	Back
Bottom of body	Top of body
Quiet	Agitation

the physical body. For example, a complete human cell is a Yin component in relation to the muscle cell that it is part of (Yang). Similarly, the muscle that was Yang in the previous example would be Yin when compared to the relationship it has with the entire arm and the muscles contained within it (Yang). Yin and Yang have to do with relationships, not absolutes.

The breath is an example of Yin and Yang. As we inhale the breath becomes Yin and as we exhale the breath becomes Yang. Our first breath when we are born is an inhalation, the Yin aspect of us becoming one the earth which is also Yin, and solidifying the union between the two. Our last breath is an exhalation, Yang, which signifies our returning to heaven.

We even see this concept in modern physics. Niels Bohr, a Danish physicist, established the science of quantum mechanics. Prior to Bohr, much debate was given to whether objects should behave as particles or waves, but not both. This science explores the essence of matter and the universe and the duel nature of reality at the subatomic level, called the principle of complementarity. Bohr's theory of waves and particles in quantum phenomena compliment each other, in other words, an object can be viewed as either a particle or a wave (Yin or Yang)! This same physical phenomenon is challenging scientists to this very day. Bohr is heralded as one of the greatest scientists of the 20th century.

In fact, even the greatest physicists today argue and debate whether light is a particle or a wave; they still cannot decide on the basic concept of light that we all see and take for granted. Simple concepts such as Qi or light from the Sun can be debated for centuries. Keep this in mind as we explore the duality of Chinese Medicine and some of its esoteric concepts.

A concept difficult for Westerners to understand Yin and Yang is ultimately about the balance of nature. Equilibrium is important in humans, animals and even plants, as is the cosmic balance of the Earth to the Sun, and galaxies to the universe. All entities have their respective place and order; one cannot change an element in one entity without affecting the other. This is the fundamental premise of Chinese medicine Yin and Yang theory.

The Five Elements

Like many indigenous cultures, the ancient Chinese use the cause and effect relations in nature to understand and map the complexities of the human body. Therefore, they used what is now called the Five Element Theory which underpins both CM and TCM. The Five Elements are Water, Wood, Fire, Earth, and Metal all moving in a clockwise pattern called the generation or production cycle. The classic definition of the production cycle is that Water causes Wood to grow, Wood gives birth or allows Fire to burn, the Fire burning produces Earth or ash or fertilizer, the Earth ash and soil then produce Metal, and the Metal through condensation produces Water, and so the cycle continues. *(See the chart)*

Out of this premise, a circular generation repesents Heaven, Earth and man. The elements are linked to seasons, to planting and harvesting, to man's health and to other attributes not thought of in western culture. The physical organs within the human body correspond to the five elements (e.g. Kidneys to Water and Heart to

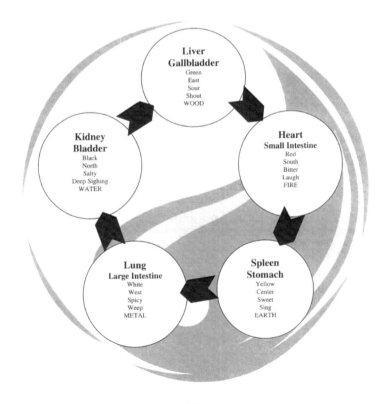

Fire) and the organs are linked to specific emotional components. This relationship of emotions to organs can then affect the Qi of the whole body leading to possibly disharmony and disease.

There is also a controlling cycle. In every successful organization there is a system of checks and balances, otherwise domination or monopoly is inevitable. Therefore, the Five Elements also control and balance one another. The following is the controlling cycle: Water controls Fire (no surprise here), Fire controls Metal (think of the making of steel or of a blacksmith), Metal controls Wood (think of a cabinetmaker and his tools), and Wood controls Earth (trees and shrubs prevent erosion) and Earth controls Water (the banks of a river or a dam).

The Taiji Pole

The Taiji pole is unique to the energetic anatomy and physiology of Taoist Chinese medicine. It is our primordial storehouse of energy and the life-force itself. It is not a physical organ, but an energetic component. Upon conception as the sperm enters the fertile egg (the first vibration and movement of life) this pole becomes activated within the first human cell and grows with us as we go through our gestation period in utero. After birth, this becomes a major transportation vessel for our very life-force or Qi and is used by the body as a reservoir of energy, a funneling system to the Three Dan tians (see below). The Taiji pole is also the very connection to the Divine or God itself.

The Taiji pole is our connection to Earth and to Heaven and is the central axis that we revolve around. It is through the Taiji pole that we remain suspended between Heaven and Earth, able to walk in the realm of the Earth but remain in the presence of the Divine or God. When connected in this way, our very core of being is vibrating (hence life itself) with the same vibration of the Divine and we commune with its very nature, while we walk on the Earth. Some refer to this ability as walking in the midst of chaos with a calm center.

The Taiji pole can be sensed or viewed by practitioners of Qigong as a brilliant white column of light piercing the darkness of the body, surrounded by golden strands of light emanating towards heaven.

The Three Dan tians

The Three Dan tians are another unique element of energetic anatomy in Chinese Medicine. The word "Dan" (pronounced "dun") translated means "cinnabar." Cinnabar was an important mineral used as a source ingredient for the production of a very special ink available only to the Chinese emperors. The word "Tian" (pronounced "t-en) means "field" or in Qigong practice, a field of energy or an orb of energy.

Qi moves through the Three Dan tians by the pathway of the Taji Pole. The Qi is then absorbed into the major organs and the tissues (i.e. muscles, tendons, ligaments, bone and skin). Additionally, there are thee regions of the human brain that also correspond to the three Dan tians. I will describe the three regions of the brain after I discuss each Dan tian in the hope that you begin to see the unique "coincidence" that the ancient Chinese could feel long before there were machines that detected these areas.

The Lower Dan tian is the most familiar of all the Dan tians. It is the storehouse of our physical strength, stamina and physical longevity. It is what most martial artists focus on in their training in order to deliver great power and force. Personal trainers and exercise physiologist speak of "training the core" when really the Chinese have been doing this for centuries.

The western correlate to the Lower Dan tian is what Michael Gershon, M.D has called "The Second Brain." In his book of the same name, he states, "The brain in the bowel has evolved in pace with the brain in the head." He is referring to the enteric nervous system, of which there are more than one hundred million nerve cells in the human small intestine alone, which rivals the amount of nerve cells in the human spinal column! If we were to take into account the other nerves from the esophagus to the large intestine, for example, we would have more nerve cells in our gut than in the entire peripheral nervous system! Something this evolved has more function than just digestion, since nature never builds and expends energy to maintain anything that does not have practical use.

Moreover, the enteric nervous system is also an enormous chemical depository containing every known neurotransmitter found in the brain itself! Neurotransmitters are the objects (i.e.waves/particles) used by nerve cells to communicate with one another and the surrounding cells. Neuroscientists are just starting to understand that the enteric nervous system and its communication links are more like the brain than any other peripheral organ. Long before the neuroscientists, Taoists priests of old understood that the Lower Dan tian is an individual, thinking, responsive system unto itself that is connected to the upper Dan tian (the brain, brain stem and spine). They empiracally devised ways of training and cultivating this energy center.

The blood-brain barrier plays an important role in such disorders as Multiple Sclerosis, brain tumors, Alzheimer's Disease, meningitis and HIV infection. This barrier, which has always baffled scientists, blocks some substances from entering the brain and allows others to enter. This barrier keeps many medications, for example drugs for cancerous brain tumors, from reaching the brain. Research at the University of Maryland has revealed that the key to the lock of the blood-brain barrier lies in the intestines! Two proteins called zonulin and zot produced in the gut provide the key to unlatch the lock in the brain! The more we find out in science, the wiser the ancients begin to appear.

The Middle Dan tian is very important to asthmatics because it contains the organs of the Heart and the Lungs. When we think of the Heart we think of blood and circulation, and of course, of the vital oxygen flowing in the blood, but CM also adds Qi to that mix. Qi and blood are inseparable. It is said in the Chinese medical classics that "Qi is the master of blood and; blood is the mother of Qi." The Middle Dan tian deals with our emotions and mental processes, including feelings which we will later see can be one of the roots of asthma attacks. Qi is also said to contain the mind and spirit (Shen in Chinese Medicine); therefore, the blood contains the mind and spirit bound by Qi.

In the early 1990's, research completed by Dr. J. Andrew Armour, a pioneer in the then new science of neurocardiology, revealed that the heart has a complex intrinsic nervous system that is quite sophisticated and evolved in its own right. In his research he refers to the "heart brain" which can act independently of the brain in the head and has its own capacity to learn, remember and even feel and sense!

Research shows that when heart rhythms are steady and oscillate with a calm, steady wave they communicate this tranquility to the brain stem (the medulla) and to the thalamus and the amygdala.

These areas link to the frontal lobes of the brain, the areas responsible for decision-making, reason and feelings, creativity and heightened mental clarity. Thus all these brain functions and states are linked to the heart! The hypothalamus, the limbic system, and the amygdala all are considered centers of emotional expression (see chart on page 39). This indicates a highly evolved communication system that we are just beginning to understand.

When you place heart cells from two different hearts in a petri dish, and keep them completely physically separated from each other, they will begin to beat with a completly new rhythm unlike each of the solitary rhythms that they previously had. This shows a very adaptive, dare I say, learned, form of energy transmission completely unseen by the naked eye. The Middle Dan tian and the heart have the power to communicate with and to influence surrounding tissues.

Additionally Dr. Candace Pert, a researcher for the National Institutes of Health, states in a 1985 paper, "Neuropeptides and their receptors…join the brain, glands and immune system in a network of communication between brain and body, probably representing the biochemical substrate of emotion." Neuropeptides are informational substances secreted by neurons (impulse conducting cells in the brain, spinal column and nerves) and lymphocytes and monocytes (both immune modulating cells in the blood). In other words, "little bits of brain" float all through the body and influence it directly. Additionally, neurotransmitters found in the brain have also been identified in the heart!

But perhaps the most convincing evidence of communication between the Middle and Upper Dan tian, or the heart and the brain, is the discovery of ANF. ANF is a hormone that is produced when the upper chambers of the heart contract (the atria). This peptide communicates with the hypothalamus and the pineal gland and influences the thalamus and the pituitary gland. What this means in English is that your emotional state, your sleep/wake cycle and your energy are all influenced by this chemical produced in the heart. Incidentally ANF affects the three regions of the brain like the three regions of the Dan tian! So what we think about in our cerebral cortex, for instance our own self induced stress, can affect the heart and the rest of the body, a three way loop of sorts. Could there be a connection here also?

Neuropeptides are so heavily influenced by stress that even under moderate stress, they shut down their automatic response process to a few minimal feedback loops, which causes a reduction in normal healing processes. Dr. Pert, who is a huge proponent of meditation, stated, "Meditation, by allowing long-buried thoughts and feelings to surface, is a way of getting the peptides flowing again, returning the body, and the emotions to health".

The Upper Dan tian is the field that represents humankind's spirituality and connection to the Divine (the top of the Taji pole). This link opens the ongoing debate of faith and medicine; can they be mixed? Is prayer effective in the healing process? What about faith in the healing process? Western science is currently trying very hard not to go there, but the lines of delineation are becoming increasingly blurred with the advent of stem cell research, human cloning, mind-body research, and prayer and medicine investigations.

The ancient Chinese based their medical systems first on energetics (bioenergy). But the Chinese, as well as many other indigenous cultures, believed that medicine and faith needed to merge. Belief was neccessary to succeed in life and to deal with the inevitable outcome of disease and death. I don't know of one person in history who ever escaped this fact of disease and death. Faith is not something you factor out in a calculus equation to prove or disprove. It is not tangible, it is not logical. Much like love, it does not depend on logic, nor does it need proof. The very fact that one has to prove that it exists negates its very action potential. Faith is destroyed by a lack of trust, which breeds doubt and failure. Ask any entrepreneur who was successful if he or she had faith in what they where doing.

A quote by Edward Teller sums it up: " When you get to the end of all the light you know and it's time to step into the darkness of the unknown, faith is knowing that one of two things will happen; either you will be given something solid to stand on, or you will be taught how to fly."

Wei chi Fields

Understanding the Qigong concept of the Wei chi (pronounced whey chee) field can be enormous help to people who suffer from allergies and asthma. The Wei chi field, for lack of better description, is a force field that exudes out from our body and surrounds us in three distinct layers. It also connects to our outer environment. The Chinese can be translated as "protective field." Schools of traditional TCM and the teachings of Medical Qigong differ in their understanding of the Wei chi field. The TCM schools believe that the Wei chi is limited to the surface of the body, and that it circulates only within the skin and the muscles. However, in Medical Qigong Chinese Medicine (CM) we believe that these fields extend beyond the body and into three external layers of auric and subtle energy that 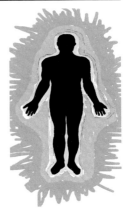 connect to the three Dan tians. Not only does the Wei chi field connect energetically to the internal organs and radiate outwardly to the external tissue of the body, but it interacts and communicates with the external environment, and most importantly for us, protects us from the pathogens of the outside world. German researchers have already identified a natural antibiotic, named Demcidin, which is secreted in sweat and is the first barrier of defense against bacteria and fungi, a natural fluid form of the inner Wei chi field.

Interestingly enough, not only can external pathogens affect us, but the inner world of our emotions or internal pathogenic factors can and will affect us as well. The world of psychology now enters into the pathology of disease because suppressed emotions such as anger or grief energetically attack our defensive Wei chi, and actually create holes in the energetic matrix.

When individuals elicite the fight, fright, or flight response (see Chapter 9), often where they will physically notice sensation is in the chest area. Tightness in the chest, tension in the neck, rapid or shallow breathing, all are communication signals from the Middle Dan tian. Remember, energy can never be destroyed, it just takes on different forms. The emotional charge (energy) if not released, must find an outlet.

Molly Barnes, M.D. found in a unique study at the University of Wisconsin that women who were sexually abused as children are more likely to develop fibromyalgia as adults. Additional studies have shown that 80% of women with chronic pain syndromes had suffered major childhood trauma. Dr. Barnes' theory is that emotional trauma creates abnormal nerve pathways that interfere with everything from heart rate to pain perception.

Prior to the human body constructing something like abnormal nerve pathways, there must be a template, a schematic drawing depicting these pathways and the trajectory of this energy. Trauma (a high emotional charge) creates the need for an emotional blueprint to be drawn, especially if this trauma is repeated. The archetect that draws the emotional blueprint in the Wei Chi and the tissues of the body is the Middle Dan tian.

Since these emotional pathogens (excessive emotional states) are vibrationally powerful (in the form of waves), they have easy access to our internal organs. The external holes created by emotions then allow pathogenic factors (virus, bacteria, fungi, etc) to burrow into the body, and these factors can manifest in a multitudes of ways. Since the linkage of the Wei Chi to the internal organs is part of the physiology of Chinese Medicine, such a degradation of the Wei Chi field and consequent invasion of pathogens can begin the state of imbalance and create disease.

The concept of an invisible form of energy emanating from the body but affecting the body physically, emotionally and perhaps spiritually as a giant biofeedback loop brings to mind an experiment performed in 1993 by the United States Army Intelligence and Security Command. White blood cells were scraped from the inside of a volunteer cheek, and placed in a test tube which was then placed in a centrifuge. Then a polygraph probe was inserted into the test tube containing the white blood cells. The volunteer later was seated in a room down the hall where he was subjected to violent scenes of fighting and killing on a television set. What is fascinating is that while the volunteer watched the carnage, the probe in the test tube recorded extreme excitation in the cheek cells even though a hallway separated the subject from his cells! Even more amazing was this experiment was repeated several times with the same result as researchers gradually increased the distance between the subject and the cells by up to fifty miles! The cheek cells remained energetically and nonlocally "connected" with their donor and his instantaneous emotional reactions. Perhaps this explains how Wei chi fields can exist as well or why certain emotions can be felt between people separated by distance.

Using meditation and Qigong exercise to strengthen the Wei chi fields helps asthmatics repulse external pathogens that may cause or exacerbate their attacks. Later, I will show how to disperse negative emotional charges and prevent them from accumulating in the Middle Dan tian.

Fear and the Kidneys

The Seven Emotion Theory In Chinese Medicine states that emotions have an energy source that can manifest into physical symtoms. This becomes clear when we think of the way emotions cause physiological changes in our bodies in the chemical realm (adrenaline rush) and the way emotions can manifest in the physical realm (breaking out in hives from nervousness). Think of how you usally come down with a cold or flu after a a time of stress. In Chinese Medicine, we believe that emotions are a normal process of living, but like anything else if accumulated in excess can lead to imbalance and potential problems such as disease. The Seven Emotion Theory linked with the Five Element Theory serve to link mind and body together in Chinese Medicine diagnoses.

We know that emotional response exacerbates hyperventilation and/or breathing disorders, and Chinese Medicine offers an eloquently explaination of the process. Since in Chinese Medicine the Lungs and the Kidneys must communicate for respiration to occur - with the Lungs controlling exhalation (Carbon Dioxide) and the Kidneys controlling inhalation (oxygen) and the movement of fluids - the rapport between them is imperative for respiration to be balanced.

Fear (Kong) is one of the Five Minds (Wu Zhi) that can promote disease process in Chinese Medicine; the other four are Shock (or excessive Excitment), Anger, Anxiety, and Thought. Constant Fear, more specifically the fear of the unknown (when is the next attack going to occur or how bad will this current attack be), and the associated excess Thought (worry) fear promotes can lead to exacerbation of the Heat in the organs. This cascade of emotions (neuropeptides) injures the Kidneys and thereby upsets the Yin/Yang balance of respiration. This constant threat that one might be unable to breathe creates Fear and results in a pathogeneses of Anxiety, which in Chinese Medicine ascends and affects the Heart (pulse rate). This syndrome, most commonly called fight, fright or flight in the West, is associated with high levels of stress or high cortisol levels.

With a chronic asthma sufferer, the Lungs are potentially already weakened, and thereby unable to disperse and lower fluids from the Spleen (digestion and assimilation); the Spleen, affected by chronic worry (of impending attacks) is unable to transform fluids; and the Kidneys, affected through chronic fear; all produce Phlegm, specifically, Substantial Phlegm or Phlegm with substance in the Lungs.

The Fear Factor and Asthma

One of the least discussed elements of chronic asthma sufferers is the fear factor, which, as the previous example suggests, latent physiological arousal. This fear factor involves two distinct responses: 1) the obvious fear generated when anyone experiences breathlessness for extended periods of time and 2) the premonition of an ominous asthma attack about to happen in certain anticipated scenarios. These two stress factors set the client up for hyperventilation as well as constriction of the very muscles used in ventilation, which further compounds the nature and progression of the asthma attack. The undeniable facts that asthma can strike during sleep, play, work, vacation, sex and in the hospital itself, makes this disease very frightening to anyone who suffers chronically.

I have worked with The American Lung Association and most recently The American Respiratory Alliance, two very proactive and vigilant groups, to educate about the prevention and treatment of asthma and other breathing disorders. This partnership allows me the opportunity to talk to and interact with thousands of asthmatics of all ages, environments, financial and educational levels. One common denominator that transcends all these differences is the fear factor. The fear factor does not discriminate on any level and can strike without even conscious warning.

As sentient beings we are the sum of our experiences. The repetitive nature of asthma attacks can be debilitating, especially since we have no direct means of actually controlling when, where or how they strike. This can cause what psychologists call learned helplessness, and this learned fear becomes our own demise. This is why Asthma Qigong, with its self-empowering nature should be a part of every asthmatic's tool kit for asthma management.

A case in point is a client of mine, a registered nurse who works in cardiovascular rehabilitation, who just happens to be an asthmatic. She becomes very nervous when exercising without her inhalater near her to the point of obsession. Her fear factor is an increasingly common one since the emergence of rescue medication like Salbutamol (Ventolin, Asmol). Although these drugs save lives, they have created a new problem. People become heavily emotionlly reliant on the drug, and the lack of its convenient presence becomes a catalyst for panic and hyperventilation leading to the self-fulfilling prophecy of an asthma attack. This is a common occurrence with my client who, despite her level of education and experience, without her inhalator in hand becomes obsessed with its absence and predictably hyperventilates into labored breathing. In this way fear is a self-fulfilling prophecy and an asthma attack is born.

Exacerbation of the Po residing in the Lungs

Several thousand years before the effects of stress were documented, the Chinese used metaphorical spirits (i.e. could not be seen) called the Po to explain how stress works on the human body. The Chinese named things as we do in an attempt to further understand something that was not tangible to the naked eye or senses, but that could definitely be felt and experienced in the body. Chinese medicine explains that the Earth-based (created by man) Po who reside in the Lungs and manifest themselves as they move through the body as Jing (essence), can be easily excited, and their animal nature may cause the exacerbation of an asthma attack by eliciting the fight, fright or flight concept.

The Po have an animalistic nature. The animal nature of the Po is to survive and to protect at any cost, (self-preservation), but they are demanding and in this way can generate negative thoughts and emotions. The seven Po "rise up", or inflame, and can be felt during the time of the asthma attack itself. In children for example, the negative thoughts of "I can't play sports or run like other kids" - further leading to thoughts of sadness or even crying because of being "different". I hear this often in talking with children at asthma camps.

Incidentally, when the military trains its special forces for survival skills, it is training the Po; when martial artists train to protect themselves, they are training the Po; when police officers do reality based training, they are training the Po; when marathon runners push past the wall of pain, they are training the Po. Like other mechanisms in the body - stress, fight, fright and flight the

Po have an important purpose and should not be thought of as "bad". They are a vehicle to save our lives when need be; we just need to learn how to harness this power correctly.

On the other hand, a more heavenly oriented set of spirits, the Hun, are what priests and holy men/women seek for enlightenment. Like all aspects of Chinese Medicine, a Yin and Yang balance is what we desire to cultivate between these two metaphorical entities.

During Asthma Qigong, the very residence of the Po (the Lungs) is addressed and calmed down, which returns the Po to a tranquil state and allows the Hun to have audience again. Understanding the nature of the Po, their location, and the visualization techniques that can be used to calm them down becomes a critical factor in our future Qigong practice.

CHAPTER 13
QiGong Exercise

QiGong, is an important tool that I believe every asthmatic should know about. Qi, as we have learned means "life energy" and gong means "life's work." So obviously we are in for a long committed length of practice here. QiGong is probably the most advanced and complete set of mind-body healing breath exercises that has ever been developed. As you study the various ways to breath, visualize, and physically control your body's movements and the Qi flow through the meridian system while in a constant state of peace of mind, you gain an enormous proactive (rather than reactive) ability to take charge of your life. Young and old, athletic and feeble, beginner and advanced can all be challenged and fulfilled with QiGong.

QiGong is really this...movement of the primordial, basic constitute of life...Qi. When we have the ability to move our Qi, then things will begin to manifest themselves in the outward body. As with life, many of the absolute truths are simple and uncomplicated. In fact, one might say that the further from the truth we get, the more tangled and twisted we become. Think of the last little fib that you told. That little fib required a lot of energy to support itself from collapsing; it began to take a life of its own after awhile. Being of a truth does not make it easy to practice or replicate however. Ask anyone who has just tried to eat less and move more to lose weight.

Here is one truth that I think we all can agree upon: Life consists of movement ...and death is the cessation of all movement. In other words, to move constitutes life in its simplest form. Movement occurs in all life, from the planets rotating around the sun, to the baby kicking in the womb, to electrons moving in the shells of an atom. Movement also creates change, most times subtly manifesting from the inside to the outside where it then becomes noticeable. Think of a chemical reaction between, say, iron and oxygen. First the movement of the electrons between the two elements interact to begin a series of changes at the atomic level. Later the two elements begin to show signs of what we call rust! For change to take place, movement must take place first originating from the inside and then gradually beginning to show itself to the outside world. This is what happens when we lose weight from the burning of calories. We just have to be patient enough for things to happen in a natural way. QiGong is the intentional moving of our life essence from which all things resonate, including our reality and perception.

Why QiGong Exercise?

As one of the oldest forms of healing, QiGong is the ultimate method of self-care I have ever found, not just for asthma, but also for a whole plethora of diseases and afflictions. Stress reduction techniques, meditation, visualization, physical therapy, occupational therapy, are only a few of it components. Every asthmatic should learn how to do these techniques as part of their survival kit. Make sure that you find a qualified teacher to guide you, because the wrong teacher will not only hinder your results, but may cause you to quit altogether from lack of results.

I think we can all agree that a massage on tired and aching muscles feels incredibly good. I can remember a time in hospitals when the night nurse would ask you if you wanted a back-rub! Gone are those days! QiGong can be likened to an internal massage for the internal organs and tissues. It should feel good, revive and kick-start you, and allow you to become more in tune with your body.

Proof of QiGong Effectiveness

QiGong is the perfect balance of movement and breathing as it is regulated by the mind's intention. Its medical applications are historically proven. Again, my definition of "proven" may be different than most, but to me for something to be proven, it must stand the test of time. For it to stand the test of time, it first has to have functionality and worth; otherwise it will be cast aside. Second, if the therapy does harm or even worse kills someone, it will no longer be passed from generation to generation. On the other hand, think of all the indigenous tribes who have encyclopedias of valuable plant and herbal preparations stored in their minds. Scientists are racing to understand this wealth of information before it is lost forever.

Even for a modern procedure or drug to be deemed safe, it has to stand the test of time. To be "proven", the procedure/drug must remain in demand and remain free from serious recalls and contraindications. It must prove itself with the Hippocratic oath in mind of "First do no harm". A drug that passes time trials for 20 or 30 years without being recalled or having warning labels attached to it is considered safe. Think of all the prematurely released pharmaceutical drugs that have later become the subject of lawsuits because they caused pain and suffering.

On prerequisites of being proven, QiGong measures up in all of these areas. QiGong, or the practice of QiGong from dated records has been around for almost 5,000 years. The actual term QiGong is relatively new, just coined in 1915 by an article where it "designates the force issued by working with the Qi and the martial applications [of this force]". [1] The practice of QiGong though, is deeply entrenched in Chinese Medicine and Taoist concepts.

Today QiGong is widely practiced under various names in China and many other countries. QiGong is Chinese in origin and in the parks of China, thousands of people practice this ancient art every day. There are roughly over 3,000 styles of QiGong in existence today. Intelligent QiGong, Five Element QiGong, Crane QiGong, Buddhist Palm QiGong, etc., are commonly practiced in QiGong circles, but most of these are QiGong for health, and not Medical QiGong, a branch of ancient Chinese Medicine.

Health Benefits

We may have heard of QiGong's very close offshoot, Tai chi chuan. Tai chi chuan is practiced in hospitals here in the United States and even has been adopted by many HMO's and outreach programs for preventative health benefits. Tai chi chuan and its mother, QiGong, have been known for their ability to reduce blood pressure, and stress, increase leg strength, reduce the risk of osteoporosis, and increase proprioception to reduce the chance of the elderly falling.

One of the most important by products of regular Tai chi chuan / QiGong practice is that it reduces the stress response. Remember that the stress response is the flight, fright or fight that we all go through when we perceive a danger, threat, or get angry, regardless of whether the threat is real or just in our mind (such as in the case of a chronic worrier or a bad dream). In the American Journal of Psychosomatic Research, stated that not only does Tai chi chuan / QiGong reduce stress (who doesn't need that these days), but it also lowers anxiety, depression, fatigue and general mood disturbances! Think of the implications of this study!

For people who are exercise-compromised, Tai chi chuan / QiGong can improve posture control while stretching, toning and relaxing the body in a cumulative way that no other form of exercise can achieve [2]. Not only that, but Tai chi chuan / QiGong is the lowest weight bearing exercise that can be performed with benefit, and modified forms can be suitable for even arthritis sufferers who can do it with only minimal discomfort [3].

Since QiGong is a Chinese practice that the West has only recently even considered a viable medical practice, we must turn to China for research and evidence that QiGong is a proven therapy for asthma, disease and health improvement.

Hospitals in China have been testing the effectiveness of QiGong for over 40 years. The effective rate in one study running statistics for over 10 years showed that QiGong was effective in 93.9% of the cases in chronic bronchial asthma.

In another study, where the average age was 64 and many of the study's participants had smoked for over 20 years, the forced vital capacity (a measurement of the lungs' ability to emit air) increased by 16.11% on average within an 18 month period. The group practiced QiGong and Tai chi chuan 3 times a week as their therapy. Six of the individuals were abnormal in Total Lung Capacity (TLC) before starting the therapy and four of them were in respiratory rehabilitation. All patients stabilized and became normal with an increase in TLC averaging 7.34%!

QiGong Meets Western Exercise Science and Rehabilitation

Western medicine and exercise science provides tools to help us understand what is truly happening in QiGong practice. It is my wish that by demystifying QiGong practice we can then see its enormous value.

Air Passages: Qigong Exercise

Let us look at a simple human movement such as normal walking at a fast pace. The arms move up and down, back and forth and slightly in front of the body; in other words they move in 3 planes of motion. Up and down, back and forth is another way of saying Yin and Yang. Multiple planes of movement involve greater amounts of neurological signaling, thereby involving more muscle tissue and creating a greater caloric burn. QiGong exercises and Tai chi chuan use multiple planes of motion in their forms.

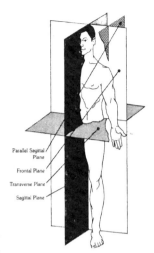

Planes of Reference

For movement to become therapeutic in nature, one must move in several planes of motion that emulate the body's natural way of moving. I recently attended a sports medicine conference whose theme was " Focus on Function." Interestingly enough, the discussion was centered on moving back to basics by training people in a somatic closed kinetic chain environment. "Somatic" means the body, "closed chain" means that both feet are on the ground, and "kinetic chain" means the mechanical forces that work on the body. In other words, use the body as resistance for rehabilitation and sport performance, rather than machines or devices. This is precisely how QiGong/Tai chi chuan works!

We can break this down further, first with Western terminology, then with Eastern. The three components of the kinetic chain are the myofascial, the articular (think of your joints) and the neural. The myofascial is a thin, translucent sheet of fibrous tissue that envelopes the body beneath the skin and separates muscle tissue. The myofascial sheet is important because when the sheet gets "kinks" in it, pain will ensue quickly.

We integrate the three components interdependently to provide optimal levels of force reduction (such as slowing the body down after a sprint or jump), stabilization (think of your joints such as knees, shoulders etc. being in control through movement), and force production (strength and explosiveness) through all three planes of motion in functional activity. Think of a football or soccer game that you recently watched as an example of the above three components.

Consider that most injuries occur in the force reduction phase (de-acceleration of the body) and around the transverse plane (see photo). Envision the transverse plane as dividing the body into top and bottom sections; that division is typically shown in anatomy books as the top of the ileum. If you are struck from behind, such as in a car accident, the body tries to stabilize itself from the force of the impact as it flies forward and then back.

Multiple planes of movement involve greater amounts of neurological signaling and therefore involve more muscle tissue. A QiGong exercise uses multiple planes of motion in its forms and movements.

So how does the Chinese Medicine concept of the Three Dan tians, QiGong and western sports medicine interrelate? The transverse plane extends through the Lower Dan tian level and is considered the center of the body. The Lower Dan tian has long been the focal point of power in martial arts and is the focus of power in Medical QiGong treatment and its therapeutic exercises! Additionally, the ming-men area (roughly L1 through L5 or the kidney area of the lower back) corresponds to the rear portion of the transverse plane. This lower region of the body is what a pro football player tries to do by dropping his "center of gravity" and driving the other person backward. On a similar note, when we hear exercise experts speak of "training the core" such as in Pilates, they are really speaking about the Lower Dan tian.

The more you can de-accelerate and stabilize the human body from the Lower Dan tian and Ming-men (or core in western therapies), the more force you can produce safely (as in sports), or recover from impact, such as an automobile accident. This is the basis of all internal martial art training (including martial QiGong). The focus is on the trunk and waist moving through a complete range of motion while stabilizing the core. Remember that a great percentage of Chinese Medicine is rooted in preventative medicine. East and West say the exact same thing only in different terminology!

The breath work involved in QiGong exercise is a critical component in making the exercises work. Knowing how to breathe efficiently (beginning with three Dan tian breathing), when to breathe, as well as how to move the breath through the various channels is the internal alchemy of QiGong exercise success. The postures allow Yin and Yang channels to open and bring Qi (energy), blood and lymphatic flow to areas that were previously deprived of healing nutrients. The movements allow Qi to flow to deeper levels and stretch the myofascial (wrapping around muscle tissue) that is many times constricted. The breath work and visualization allow the body to relax and decompress from stress, and to release restriction and muscular tightness that previously caused pain, muscular knots and discomfort. The whole time this is happening, the heart rate slows, blood pressure drops, respiration becomes deep and slow, and there is an increase of oxygen to the tissues. The body is in a state of healing similar to sleep, but mobile and active, moving healing blood and lymph through the tissues.

Working in the fitness field has allowed me to observe many types of exercises and the people performing them. I have noticed that many people in today's gyms want to be diverted from listening to their body as they are exercising. The number of headsets being used in the gym, the background noise and the loud music being played all contribute to desensitizing the mind from the body. When I visited Vince Gironda's gym in Hollywood, California many years back, he did not allow music of any kind to be played there. Vince was a trainer to many movie stars, and he believed that vivid visualization, concentration and total mental commitment were what the mind should be focused on. Try one workout without music in the quiet of your own home or a friend's gym and notice how difficult the poundage is to lift after a while. QiGong is like that. We do not want any distractions from introspecting into our bodies and listening to what it is trying to tell us as we exercise and breathe.

QiGong Applications

Unlike Tai chi chuan, QiGong exercises can be performed sitting, standing or even lying in bed. In addition, the movements are singular in nature and less like a martial arts form or kata. Unlike yoga, most postures are not held for a length of time and do not require any props or mats. Unlike Pilates, there are no machines or ropes to be utilized as part of the training. Because of its slow gentle nature, seniors who have never exercised before, the obese, or the sickly and frail, can all start QiGong exercises and participate in a full class without having to stop to rest. This ability to complete something with the rest of the class does wonders for the psyche of a client. When observed from afar the exercises do not appear intimidating at all and therefore may attract shy intimidated newcomers to begin exercising. This broad based practice can therefore be applied to a very diverse population with very different needs....the very population that may need exercise and the movement of Qi the most.

Three Branches of Qigong

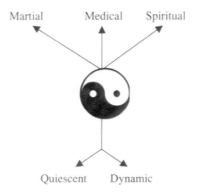

The uniqueness of QiGong exercises does not stop there. In Western terms, QiGong exercises are a combination of continuous static stretching and compound movements stabilizing the core that also combine breath-work, visualization and even sound therapy. This multi-faceted approach is indeed more progressive in its foresight of how the body works and rebuilds itself as a whole.

Simplicity always works best in nature; although the inner working and details may be overwhelming and exhaustive, the basic premise must be simple. So, too, is QiGong practice. There are two major subsets of QiGong: 1) Dynamic QiGong, or moving QiGong (dong gong); and 2) quiescent QiGong, or meditative QiGong (jing gong). Quiescent QiGong is more akin to the seated meditation poses that one can't help but see on television these days or in the movies. Within the two subsets, there are the three branches of QiGong practice: Medical, Martial and Spiritual. For example, one may practice Medical QiGong in either a moving or a outwardly still fashion.

Chinese Medical QiGong Exercise Prescription versus QiGong Exercise for Health

It is always difficult to explain what I do as a Doctor of Medical QiGong to client/patients and to western professions including physical therapy, chiropractic, massage, and of course, medical doctors. What is the difference between someone leading a group or individual through a QiGong movement form, and "prescribing" a specific exercise for a health condition?

In Chinese Medicine, there is a whole hierarchy of pathways that all are connected to every fiber of the body, although which most people are not aware of them. These pathways could be considered different levels or complete systems unto themselves rather like western medicine's circulatory and nervous systems. Like western medicine, the study and details of these internal pathways is complex. These pathways are layered and crossed and connect with the internal organs and even the emotional repositories of the body (remember in Chinese Medicine, physical, emotional and spiritual are connected).

The term for these acupuncture meridians and collaterals (or pathways) is the Jingluo. "Jing" means channel, and "Luo" (collateral) means to attach like the strands of a net across the body. The "Jing" are what a typical acupuncture chart shows and what most people are familiar with from reading about Chinese Medicine, or about striking in martial arts or about pressure point therapies. The "Luo" are cross branches that intersect the meridians. These meridian pathways contribute to exercise effectiveness, systemic health, as well as the healing of various diseases.

These meridian systems; grouped in order from the most superficial to the deepest regions of the body are: the cutaneous regions, the minute collaterals, the sinew channels, the luo-connecting channels, the primary channels, the divergent channels, the extraordinary channels, and finally the deepest pathways of the primary and divergent channels. A lot of new terms, but perhaps it will give you a perspective of how intricate the Chinese medical system is.

To prescribe a therapeutic QiGong exercise for a particular individual, the QiGong doctor must know all these levels of channels, much like a surgeon would know western anatomy to operate. In addition, the QiGong doctor must know the correct Qi flow patterns in these levels and channels. That is why Medical QiGong Doctors are considered some of the most advanced practitioners of Chinese Medicine in that they understand these systems fully.

It is believed in Chinese Medicine that an external pathogen or trauma starts at skin and hair level and burrows itself inward using this system of pathways. We look at the origin of the illness and treat from there. The depth to which the pathogen has penetrated the Jingluo indicates how serious the ailment is. We use the various depths to understand what Zangfu (the six Yin and Yang organs) the pathogen may have penetrated. Understanding this, we can plot the pathogens/trajectory and predict what organs it will next affect and how the body will react. Knowing this trajectory also helps us figure out where to start treatment. Treatment, then, is like following a flow chart backward to its origin.

The Jingluo are actually what make exercise work or not work in a rehabilitation setting. The selection and balancing of Medical QiGong exercises to the appropriate obstruction, blockage or pathogen that is causing the person pain, discomfort or lack of mobility is imperative to success. In this, QiGong prescriptions have much in common with physical therapy, occupational therapy, gait therapy, proprioception and kinesthesia. The Medical QiGong Doctor uses a variety of diagnostic tools and a diagnostic paradigm that differs from that of western medicine. So, although several people may have the same western diagnosis, eastern diagnosis may prove that each person has a different set of imbalances or invasions that can be remedied by different exercise methods.

The diagnostic tools listed here for your knowledge of their existence. Know that when you visit a Chinese Medicine practitioner, s/he will use a number of diagnostic tools. Use this list as a reference when you seek out a practitioner. Some of the more common evaluation techniques include: tongue analysis, pulse analysis, the patterns of the eight principals, the five element theory, examining the eyes and complexion and incorporating the seven emotion theory into the diagnosis. The practitioner will also ask many questions about lifestyle and habits. The practitioner will take the time to listen to and examine the client, and think about what s/he finds is in context of his/her knowledge of all the Jingluo. Then the practitioner will devise an exercise solution. As a reference, I usually meet with someone at least 2 hours on the first appointment.

For health, its maintenance, and even sports, we use a variety of positions, postures and movements that correspond to the channels, collaterals and vessels we are trying to stimulate, or to which we are trying to increase the Qi flow. The point is to facilitate the balance of structure and integrity between Yin and Yang. When Yin and Yang are balanced, then the body can work optimally in one's particular sport (even if that sport is full contact gardening) and the efficiency of that sport can improve as well as our health and immunity.

Remember that Yin and Yang refer to left and right, top and bottom, back and front, inside and outside. From the perspective of Yin and Yang, to do a full body workout you must work the whole body, not just, for example, the biceps or chest. You must both lift weight (contract or Yin), and stretch and elongate (extend or Yang). The finite balance in the human body is what we are after in QiGong exercise prescription. All QiGong exercise can be beneficial and relaxing when done properly. Medical QiGong exercise prescription is targeted specifically for an individual, based on CM or TCM diagnosis, and crafted to affect the specific Jinglou areas needed.

Chinese Medical QiGong

In a hierarchy of QiGong practice, the highest level of QiGong for health and longevity is Medical QiGong. Medical QiGong is practiced in many hospitals in China and is one of the four main branches in original Chinese Medicine. Acupuncture and herbology are probably the two most well known branches of Chinese medicine followed by Bodywork (such as Tuina) and QiGong.

In China, when no one else was able to help a particular patient, they were referred to a Doctor of Medical QiGong (DMQ). The Doctor of Medical QiGong has all the diagnostic background of say an acupuncturist or an herbalist, but they operate in a very different fashion. The DMQ does not use needles or herbs, but relies on his/her own understanding of Qi to directly move the blocked/stagnant Qi in the client.

In China, most hospitals include the practice of Medical QiGong as part of the full prescription given by doctors. For example, after applying a cast to a broken limb in an ER, the doctor would refer the patient to a DMQ. The DMQ might prescribe a QiGong exercise to promote circulation of Qi flow to heal the injury faster and with fewer complications. Many hospitals use QiGong treatments exclusively to help with everything from migraine headaches to the treatment of cancer.

Xi Yuan Medical QiGong Hospital is one of the oldest and largest research hospitals in China. Xi Yuan hospital is also a graduate teaching hospital for Medical QiGong therapy. The hospital is best known for Medical QiGong treatments in many types of cancer (especially the dissolving of tumors and cysts), Fibromyalgia, Chronic Fatigue Syndrome, coronary heart disease, asthma, gastric intestinal disease, nephropathy and many other ailments.

Many of the successful Medical QiGong physicians in China that I have met attribute their success of Medical QiGong to their continued practice of Martial QiGong and various unique meditations which help them avoid depleting their own Qi. In reality, the three branches of QiGong do merge to a certain extent as one does help promote the other.

QiGong physicians in China believe that they must be in good health to effectively treat the vast number of patients they see each day. In order to promote good health, they practice health QiGong (dynamic or quiescent or both) and martial arts. Predominately, they practice internal martial art techniques (Nei dan or internal elixir), systems such as Tai chi chuan, Pa Kua, Liu Ho Ba Fa, and Hsing Yi. The physicians also do specific and very detailed meditations for increasing the balance of Yin and Yang within their own bodies.

Distilling Chinese medicine down greatly, one could say that disease or illness arises from four components: congenital, pernicious influences, emotions, and individual lifestyle.

Congenital or genetic conditions are explained as Qi imbalances inherited by the embryo from the parents' Qi.

Pernicious influences or environment is defined as pollution of any sort. This could be a vapor from the paint on your walls to the chemicals in your carpets to dust, pollens, bacteria and viruses floating in the air. All of which would roughly translate to wind or perhaps cold invasion in Chinese Medicine.

Air Passages: Qigong Exercise

Chinese Medicine has perhaps the most comprehensive perspective of the relations between emotions and health. Chinese Emotional Theory believes that the resonance of any emotion - its energy (Qi) and the chemical reactions that emotion elicits - can greatly affect health. We often talk about how stress can cause everything from headaches to falling seriously ill, but we never consider like the Chinese do, how all the emotions together affect the body and its chemistry.

Lifestyle would be a combination of your eating, sleeping and drinking habits (from alcoholic drinks to water) and the quantity you consume of each.

The Doctor of Medical QiGong (DMQ) also uses herbs (Pa Fa) to internally treat the Qi as well, and may refer out to an herbalist. Similarly, the doctor may also choose to refer his or her patient to a qualified therapist or counselor who is willing to work with the Medical QiGong Doctor to deal with any emotional issues that may come up during treatment.

One of the greatest gifts we can give someone is to empower him or her. Children and adults both need to feel as if they have some semblance of control of their lives and can make a difference and contribute to the process of healing. The DMQ empowers the patient by allowing them to be proactive in their own health care again, rather than being at the mercy of a practitioner.

The main goal of treatment is to facilitate the alignment of Qi within the body and to clear all stagnate and congealed Qi from the meridians, vessels, and collaterals. Once that is successfully completed, the QiGong doctor then will purge or tonify the actual Zangfu organs (the six Yin and six Yang organs). The next step is to make sure that no one organ became over charged with Qi during the course of treatment.. The doctor must also check and see if Qi flows in the correct direction to corresponding Zangfu organs. If the direction of Qi is not correctly done (incorrect Qi flow may have caused disease or illness in the first place), the patient can become very ill or suffer new complications. Next, the Three Dan tians are charged and balanced. Finally, the QiGong Doctor prescribes detailed and specific "exercises" based on the findings of the session. These exercises help move, balance, tonify or purge Qi based on the specific needs of the patient. It is the patient's responsibility to practice these exercises on his or her path to good health. When the alignment of Qi is properly balanced, neither too

Air Passages: Qigong Exercise

Yin nor too Yang, we have the foundation of health and are better protected from disease.

The Medical QiGong system of health care, although almost unheard of in this country, plays a very important role in the Chinese health care system. I outline it here not to argue that it should replace western medicine, but to show what a valuable component it is. It is somewhat ironic to think that in China, Western medicine is considered "alternative" by the common people, and for many, is not quite trusted as much as their traditional system.

(1) The Way of QiGong; Kenneth S. Cohen
(2) American Journal of Occupational Therapy
(3) American Journal of Physical Medicine and Rehabilitation

CHAPTER 14
Asthma QiGong

The purpose of Asthma QiGong is to reduce the quantity and frequency of asthma attacks, reduce the amount and dose of medications needed (inhaled steroids or rescue Albuterol), return or bring an internal sense of self control to the asthmatic, and reduce the fear factor of asthma attacks.

Getting Started

Using this method, some of my clients have been able to reduce the number of asthma attacks and the frequency of using their inhalators within three weeks! In order to obtain these results, diligent study and practice is required.

There is not a traditional warm-up for QiGong exercise in the sense of western "warmups" because each movement is very slow and deliberate, and thus gently warms the exercised area. The only warm-up we do is to center the mind through breathing techniques before beginning our exercises in order to have a fruitful practice. Many clients of mine use this technique throughout their day at work or at home to counteract their feelings of becoming "overwhelmed" or stressed.

The order of QiGong exercises is not important as long as all five-Yin organs are worked in the same session. The five Yin organs of Chinese Medicine are the Kidneys, Liver, Spleen, Heart and Lungs. In Chinese medicine, when the five Yin organs are equally strong, balanced and toned, then one can enjoy robust health and longevity. Once the Yin organs are exercised, one should "blend" the energy together so that one organ is not stronger than another. Similar to making a cake, once all the ingredients are added, the batter needs to be blended smoothly and evenly. This is accomplished by performing a QiGong exercise that does not pertain to one particular organ, but works on the natural Qi flow of the body. Qi has certain pathways, like rivers in the Earth, that it follows when one is healthy. We try to emulate this natural pathway when we close our QiGong session and bring our body back to the very center from which we started.

The breath work involved in QiGong exercise is a critical component in making the exercises effective. Breathing efficiently begins with Three Dan tian breathing (three regions of breath in Chapter 4) , and knowing when to breathe, as well as how (visually) to move the breath through the various channels. This is the internal alchemy of QiGong exercise success. This breath work and visualization are key to stress reduction in that they occupy the mind so intensely that it overshadows the day's problems.

An old truth states that simple works best and is the most effective. I might add that having the right teacher can make a world of difference in whether you enjoy, understand and stick with any new course you take.

Centering

Try this exercise to center your mind or calm your thoughts down. Sit comfortably in a chair or on a bench so that your hips are higher than your knees. This brings the correct breathing posture into play for energy movement through the body. Sit with your back straight, not slouched, with your head as though you were holding up a ceiling with the soft spot on your head. Now, close your mouth and begin to inhale breath in with your nose. Feel it travel down into the lower reaches of your stomach as your back and stomach begin to expand with newfound life force being poured into the deepest lobes of your lungs. Exhale slowly out the mouth through pursed lips as if blowing up a balloon. Focus your mind to center on the area below your navel (Lower Dan tian) and imagine that area growing warm with blood and life force. Continue to breathe in this manner until you begin to slow down your rate of respiration to six breaths per minute as a goal. This can be completed anywhere, any time of the day.

Breath Ratio Breathing Methods

There are many different and complete methods of breathing in which you manipulate the variables of inhalation, exhalation and the pauses between them. In addition, whether you breathe in through your nose and exhale through your nose or exhale through your mouth can all have different effects on the body, nervous system, blood pressure and the endocrine system. For example, by lengthening and pausing after exhalation (all the air is passed out), can have a more relaxing effect. Conversely, if you lengthen and pause your inhalation, this type of breathing can energize you!

If you think about breath and the length of inhale, exhale and the pauses, and if you correlate them to musical beats or seconds, you can estimate the time required for each portion of a complete breath to take place. For example, if you inhale for 4 counts, pause for 1 count, exhale for 8 counts and then pause for 4 counts this is one complete breath cycle. This particular method will also relax you (Yin exercise) and will decrease blood pressure by stimulating the parasympathetic nervous system.

On the other hand, if you breath in for 6 counts, pause for 6 counts, exhale for 6 counts and pause for 1 count, this will energize you (Yang exercise). For a more balancing effect of Yin and Yang, you can inhale for 8 counts, pause for 1, exhale for 8, and pause for 1 count. This balanced exercise is better if you are feeling stressed, because holding breath on the inhalation can add more tension in this case.

After you have been practicing the Asthma QiGong exercises for awhile, I would recommend at some point doing what is called the windy breathing method. This method is accomplished by doing all breathing through the nose (inhale and exhale) thereby warming and filtering the air so as not to shock the body. This particular method stimulates the pituitary gland (the master gland responsible for cortisol production) by vibrating the nasal passages through constant oscillation in the nose. In Chinese Medicine the Lung energy begins with the nose, hence the focus on this area.

The Three Steps of Practice

There are only three steps that must be adhered to for your QiGong practice to be effective and healthy are:

1. Purge. Disperse the negative Qi before ingesting new fresh Qi.
2. Tonify. Work all five internal Yin (Zang) organs.
3. Blend. Balance the energy upon closing.

Before we start the purgation exercise, let me explain the posture you will be in for the remainder of the QiGong Asthma exercises.

Wuchi Posture

Wuchi posture starts with the feet a little wider than shoulder width apart with the toes pointing as close to straight ahead as comfortable. The knees are slightly bent to take pressure off the lower back. The pelvis is slightly tipped forward with the weight being felt in the front of the thighs. The spine is relaxed and so is the musculature of the body. Pretend that your head is pushing up/holding the ceiling using the crown of your head. Your chin dips slightly toward your chest. The position should feel comfortable. I always had a tendency to thrust my shoulders back and hold my chest tight. Relax the shoulders, let them "round," and allow the chest to drop a little. You will feel a connection with the ground like gravity is pulling you into the earth.

Purging

The importance of this concept was brought home to me by my teacher, Dr. Jerry Allen Johnson. He said, "if I offered you a glass of clean bottled water, you would probably welcome it if you were thirsty. Now if I poured the water into a dirty glass, would you still drink it? Probably not. Most people would not take the chance of contamination. Purging the body of negative Qi is much the same." Why would you want to put clean energy into a dirty container?

To start the purgation process, begin in the above Wuchi posture Centering yourself for a few minutes. Raise the arms up to the sides gathering all emotional turmoil that you have acquired during the day into a ball of sludge in your left hand and then rotating to the right; toss the sludge of emotional upheaval away into the air. Different emotions originate/collect in different places in Chinese Medicine. For example, jealousy occurs in the Liver on the right side of the torso, worry occurs in Spleen on the left side, fear occurs in the Kidneys, grief and despair in the Lungs, and shock and violation of social boundaries in the Heart.

You must feel and actively visualize this happening for this to work. Center yourself again and this time allow all the toxic emotional sludge to roll to your right hand; twist to the left and again toss the sludge away. Repeat this as many times as necessary for you.

Tonify the Five Yin Organs

There are five Yin organs in Chinese medicine (well, actually six but many texts do not acknowledge the Pericardium). They are the Kidneys, Liver, Spleen, Heart and Lungs. There are exercises for each of these organs; and each of these organs has influence on the other. When all organs are balanced and energized appropriately the body is strong enough to fight off pernicious (environmental conditions that cause disease) influences. We are going to place extra emphasis on the Lungs, Spleen and Kidneys, because these organs are classically the deficient organs when it comes to allergies and asthma in Chinese Medicine. Extra emphasis on these organs will bring the body back to balance from its inherent weakness.

Preparation for Working the Yin Organs

Before we start, let us connect the Yin and Yang channels in the body and seal the vessel of the torso. This is a must in true QiGong practice in order to keep the energy we acquire. Place your tongue behind your upper teeth, lightly touching the soft upper palate. The tongue position will vary depending on the organ we are working with. Contract the muscle that controls the perineum, which is located between the genitalia and the anus. This is the portal that allows the Qi to be stored in the upper Yin organs and the three Dan tians. Think of this as a "cork" that seals the energy from "running out," like a stopper that keeps bath water from running down the drain of a bathtub.

Pull Down the Heavens QiGong Exercise:

Inhale slowly and deeply with the palms of the hands facing the Yin of the Earth. Slowly raise the hands (palms facing down) above the head while expanding the lungs. Feel the Qi flow deeply into the lower Dan tian and expanding outward into the six directions of Qi (front and back, left and right, top and bottom). This is sometimes called Wen Huo breathing in QiGong. To illustrate filling the lungs with air/Qi, in your mind, envision holding an empty balloon in front of you and slowly filling it with water. You will notice at first the balloon drops toward Earth with the weight of the water, but as the balloon starts to fill, it gradually expands evenly in all directions.

Exhale and with the palms now facing upward towards heaven, begin to pull the Yang energy of Heaven into the Taji pole moving through all three Dan tians. Pull and condense the Qi into the Lower Dan tian by contracting inward (opposite six directions of Qi), which is natural while exhaling as the diaphragm expands upwards and pushes the air out. Feel the Qi becoming brighter and glowing in the lower Dan tian. This is one complete cycle. Perform this cycle 36 times in a row.

A Reminder: Use the balancing technique of breath ratio's to start. Once you are comfortable with the QiGong exercises, do all of the following with the windy breathing method one time per day. For additional daily practice, you can perform the long exhalation technique for relaxing, calming and lowering blood pressure (Yin exercise).

QiGong Lung Exercise

After centering yourself in Wuchi posture, place the tongue between the teeth of the upper and lower jaw and, begin by rubbing your palms together faster and faster until you feel heat building up in the palms. Once they are nice and warm, quickly place your hands on your chest at nipple level, inhale deeply and suck in and absorb the heat from the palms deep into the chest. Feel the heat penetrate the smallest space of your lungs as it thins and melts away the mucous inside the lung tissue. Inhale the heat several times, bringing it deeper and deeper into the lung cavity. Once there is no more heat to absorb, mentally circulate the heat through the chest, further thinning the mucous and then draining the mucous down into the bowels (Large Intestine) to be later excreted. Visualize swirling water through a stained jar and then dumping the turbid water down the drain into the sink, leaving the jar clean and sparkling. After this, inhale; open the arms wide (parallel to the shoulders) with your palms down pulling clean energy from the earth into the palms of the hands. Pull this energy into your lung tissue enveloping the bronchiole tubes while you open and expand them with Qi. As you exhale, move the palms upwards towards the sky, like a bellows releasing all the inflammation toward heaven. Bring the arms together in front of the chest. Repeat this movement 9 times in a row. Remember that the true link between mind and body begins and ends with the breath. Learn to control the breath and the pause between the breath and you will learn to control this vital link.

Additionally, you can perform a sound or tone that sounds like "shhhhhh" on the exhale. This is a Medical QiGong technique to additionally purge stagnation in the Lungs as well.

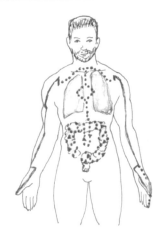

Interrelationship of the Lung meridian and the Large Intestine meridian.

QiGong Spleen Exercise

The spleen exercise is designed to "open" the spaces of the Spleen not only from an energetic channel point of view, but in terms of Western anatomy and physiology. Have someone watch your posture, or videotape yourself to pick out tightness, tension and inconsistencies from left to right, and front to back when observing yourself for postural asthma. Someone with hunched shoulders and rounded upper torso with hypertrophied neck muscles is usually a good candidate for a Spleen exercise.

Start in Wuchi again and center yourself. Begin by inhaling deeply, bring the arms to waist height and then move them towards each other in back of you, forming a triangle with both hands meeting behind the back about hip height. Bring the tongue to rest on the bottom on the mouth and curl it under. Depress the shoulders and the shoulder blades downward so that you feel a mild stretch in the rib cage as you expand your chest area upward. You are still doing abdominal breathing; keep the head upright as if supporting the ceiling with the soft spot on your head. Inhale energy up the inside of the legs, through the hips into the large area of the chest (around nipple level). Turn your head to the left as you rotate to the left while pulling the triangle of the hands slightly down and out in the opposite direction. You should feel a stretch in the oblique muscles and the waist area. While exhaling, purge through the mouth all the dampness and wind from the body that can be the cause of asthma and allergies. Return to the front and exhale through the mouth. Repeat on the right side. Perform 9 repetitions.

QiGong Kidney Exercise

It is interesting to note that recent scientific discoveries by Western medicine confirm the existence of a relationship between the Lung and the Kidney that was deduced by Medical QiGong Doctors centuries ago. The kidneys produce a hormone called erythropoietin that becomes available to the body when the blood oxygen levels are low. This hormone then signals the body to deposit more red blood cells into circulation and therefore more hemoglobin, which carries the oxygen. Since there is more taxi service so to speak, the greater the possibility that what limited oxygen is available will get transported to where it is needed. Homeostasis is achieved again by the miraculous communication between the kidneys and the lungs. Modern science is catching up to the wondrous knowledge of QiGong!

In ancient China the Kidneys were called the lotus bulbs. The Chinese believed that from the Kidneys grew the spinal column called the lotus stem and ended with the lotus flower called the brain.

Begin this exercise by placing the tongue on the soft palate at the back of the upper palate while centering yourself. Start by rubbing your hands together until hot from friction. Place them on your back, covering the Kidneys and inhale, drawing the heat in the Kidneys for 9 full (inhale/exhale) breaths. Next rotate from the waist in a clockwise direction, still drawing in the energy from the hands for another 9 breaths. Do this slowly and deliberately and time the rotation so as to inhale while bending back and exhale while coming forward. Finally, rotate in counterclockwise direction for 9 breaths in the same fashion.

QiGong Heart Exercise

Begin by placing the tongue softly against the upper palate as before in a Wuchi posture. Step forward in a lunge position with the left leg, while circling the arms in front of your chest as if grabbing hold of a large barrel. The left hand positioned at the heart level will pull energy into the Heart/ Pericardium area, while the right hand placed near the right hip pulls energy in from the Earth. Come back to Wuchi and repeat on the other side for a total of 9 repetitions each side.

QiGong Liver Exercise

The Liver exercise is the only exercise that we classically do as purgation. The reason is that the Liver contains all the frustration, anger and jealousy that we acquire in a stress filled day. For that reason, we will do a purgation movement for this Yin organ.

Start by opening the perineum since we want to drain the Liver energy, and dropping the tongue to the bottom of the mouth along the lower gumline. Step out from Wuchi posture and begin by placing the left hand outstretched in front of the body as if punching, but with an open palm. The right hand is back along the Liver organ itself, against the lower ribs. While alternating the arms in a punching/palm position, breath one inhalation for every three movements of the left and right hands. Pause the breath, and then exhale for another 3 movements of the left and right hands. Repeat for a total of 9 repetitions.

Blend

Blending the Qi flow throughout the meridians, the organs, and the vessels is the final step of QiGong practice. This is analogous to filling an ice cube tray: one compartment may have too little water, one too much, and none are equal in the quantity of water they hold. Before placing the tray in the freezer as it were, we do a simple QiGong exercise of tipping the tray to bring uniformity to the compartments of the tray, so that there is balance again. This is like the Qi in the body; we must, before closing the door, equal out the Qi in the body's compartments so that balance/health is restored. Otherwise, we can create a condition equal or worse to the one that we are trying to fix. This all begins with a concept in Chinese Medicine called the microcosmic orbit.

Microcosmic orbit

The microcosmic orbit is the ultimate way to blend the cultivated Qi from your QiGong practice and "smooth" it out throughout the body. Similar to baking a cake, you have just entered the ingredients into the pan (the Lungs, Spleen, Kidney, Heart and Liver exercises); now we must mix them up evenly in the body, like blending the cake batter together and smoothing out the top of the pan. The exercise itself is actually a combination of movement/breath and intention. It was kept secret to many practitioners until the last 20 years or so. The idea was that without this vital link the concepts and benefits of Chinese medicine would elude most practitioners. I can vouch for this myself as many martial arts instructors would allude to knowing this and other concepts, but would never elaborate on the details.

Again begin in the Wuchi posture. Connect the Yin and Yang channels in the body and seal the vessel of the torso. Place your tongue behind your upper teeth, lightly touching the upper palate. Contract the muscle that controls the perineum, which is located between the genitalia and the anus. Remember, this is the portal that allows the Qi to be stored in the upper Yin organs and the three Dan tians. Don't forget that this seals the energy from "running out", like a stopper.

Once this posture is comfortable, feel your feet "melt" into the earth and become one with the elements of nature. Inhale, feel warm energy rush up the legs from the earth like an artesian well spouting water. Let this water-like feeling continue up the upper thighs, up the back via the spine and rush over the top of the head. On the exhalation, feel the warm water continue down the front of the face, to the chin, the upper chest, and on down to the lower Dan tian, where the energy is stored like a huge lake of Qi. The energy coming up the back will feel like a fire hydrant gushing, and the descent of energy in the front of the body will feel like a heavy rainstorm flowing over the body.

The above description is the Yang aspect of the microcosmic orbit or the male version. Women (Yin) need to reverse the flow by allowing energy to flow up the front and then down the back. I have seen incredible results in women who use this method (water method) rather than the male (fire) method. This was confirmed by my Taoist teacher, an 88th generation priest and Chinese doctor, who states that the microcosmic orbit is opposite for women than for men. Many QiGong teachers will tell you otherwise, but they are misinformed. QiGong was traditionally a male practice. Male teachers passed it to male students generation after generation, and in this way the proper direction for women's microcosmic orbit became lost. The truth needs to be explained now since more and more women are doing QiGong.

Additionally, do not worry about when to inhale or when to exhale. Relax, feel the energy, inhale deeply and exhale deeply. Repeat this process from the legs up. Once you are comfortable with the visualization part of this, and it becomes natural, you can really enjoy the benefits of this exercise. This will lull you into a meditative state like nothing else I have ever tried.

Do not be alarmed if you feel warmth, tingling and even heat coming from your lower Dan tian, as this is the energy building in your core. This exercise is the basis of your Qi being healthy and in turn, you being healthy. You can continue this exercise for the rest of your life and continue to reap the benefits from it.

Kwon Kong Stroking Beard

This exercise is very old and utilizes what we have learned in the microcosmic orbit practice. Using the hands to direct the Qi, inhale and begin by moving the hands slowly up the torso while visualizing the artesian well spouting water up the back. The hands keeping pace with the flow of energy, slowly lead Qi up to the top of the head on the inhalation. As the energy crests the top of the head, exhale and feel the clean energy fall over the eyes and nose like a mighty waterfall. Synchronize your hands and your breathe to the movement of the Qi, bring them back down the front of the torso and let them come to rest at the Lower Dan tian. Repeat 100 times. Make sure that you *feel* this practice rather than just go through the mechanics of it. Remember ladies your version is reverse of this description. Finish Kwon Kong by Pulling Down the Heavens three times.

This will conclude your QiGong practice session.

Asthma QiGong Preventative Maintenance Program

QiGong exercises are one of the most powerful and integrated therapies man has yet devised for his own health and well-being. It does not take any equipment, is portable and can be performed anywhere. Asthma QiGong for preventative maintenance should be done several times per day in order to stabilize the pH of the body and to prevent hyperventilation and other incorrect breathing patterns. The structured reprogramming of the nervous system is what the practitioner is achieving. The nervous system, as defined by Dr. John Shen, is responsible for the central and peripheral pathways controlling the smooth muscle tissues (autonomic nervous system), the musculoskeletal systems as well as Kidney – Jing essence and the sea of marrow (spinal column and brain); more specifically the neurological feedback loop ushering impulses to the brain itself.

Preventative maintenance should be a staple of living for the asthmatic patient, much like bathing, sleeping and eating are deemed necessary. The methods described here should be practiced daily as a means to acquaint the mind with a sense of comfort and neurological patternization that will allow the you to slip into the state of relaxation response.

The basic premise of all of these exercises is to focus the Shen (mind/intent/spirit) into the organs and to visualize the energy flowing into the channels, as it clears out the phlegm and inflammation of the lung tissue and purges this energy out through the anus. Most phlegm and mucous naturally drain into the stomach when we swallow or are congested, especially at night, later excreted through the colon or large intestine and finally out the anus. Since the Lungs and the Large Intestine are paired organs in Chinese Medicine, the anus is a natural destination for toxic pathogenic factors that the body needs to purge.

The goal is to bring the respiration rate down to six complete breaths per minute or one complete inhale/ pause exhale/pause cycle every ten seconds. It is interesting to note that all chants regardless of dogma or culture, work on this 10-second premise of time through spacing of breath and words. Additionally, many osteopaths using cranial sacral therapy also notice a rhythm of six to twelve cycles per minute between the pulse of the cranium and sacrum.

Since the elemental nature of asthma deals with the Lungs, Kidneys, and Spleen, all Yin organs, we need to work on the number of respirations completed per daily prescription.

The best time to practice Asthma QiGong is between the hours of 3 and 5 pm. For those of us familiar with Chinese medicine that is not surprising, as that is when the Lungs are furthest from their peak of energetic Qi saturation (3-5 am) and more open to absorbing Qi from QiGong practice. However, when western research scientists "discovered" that corticosteroids, whether inhaled or administered orally, were most effective in controlling asthma symptoms when administered at 3pm, they confirmed what the ancients knew all along, that Qi, can best be absorbed by the Lungs. This was actually researched earlier by an Italian pharmaceutical company that conditionally prescribed their asthma medication to be taken at 3pm in the afternoon. All of their research confirms the natural clock of the human body outlined in the classic writings of Chinese medicine.

It may seem like these exercises take a lot of effort or take too much time in their need to be done consistently. Nothing, however, can compare to the reward of taking back control of your own life, eliminating your worst fear(s), and empowering yourself towards your true potential. Focus on these positive attributes, and I am certain that you will look forward to your training time as an investment in yourself.

CHAPTER 15
Chinese Herbals

Many herbals that I like to use to manage asthma and allergies come from China. Some of these formulas are customized, others are standard formulas used throughout the world. The standardized formulas are called patent medicines in China and are hundreds, or sometimes thousands, of years old. Many of the original formulae go back to the Shaolin temple and beyond. In fact, the first Materia Medica (a kind of a physician's desk reference for herbalists), was written by the Chinese herbalist Shen Nong around 2838 B.C and was called the *Sheng Nong Ben Cao*.

A patent medicine works on the premise that the sum of the parts strengthens the whole. In other words, various herbs are used synergistically. They combine to form a unique chemical compound different from the original properties of the various ingredients. Today the Materia Medica of Chinese medicine contains over 5,000 substances that all can be combined in multiple ways depending on the objective of the herbalist.

Chinese herbalism also uses mushrooms, lizards, snails, deer antlers and other very esoteric ingredients to formulate these unique chemical compounds. What is truly amazing is that all of these substances have been researched for their properties and effects and classified into Yin and Yang, ascending or descending, warm and cool etc.

As any good doctor, the herbalist selects from the information he has gathered from the client or patient and decides on a desired course of events designed to produce a final outcome. The Chinese Materia Medica assembles possible outcomes into at least 18 groupings. These desired outcome may sound strange to the western ear. Herbs can be, for example, blood rectifying, exterior resolving, wind dispelling, liver calming and phlegm transforming. From the Materia Medica the herbalist would choose ingredients that will support the desired final outcome based on groupings he or she has deemed worthwhile. The herbalist may choose to do this in several stages so the transformation the herbs will induce will not overwhelm the body or the client.

As stated before, Chinese Medicine adopts the viewpoint of asthma is not just about the Lungs, but about the Spleen and the Kidneys as well. The root cause that is being diagnosed is a complex issue to resolve, as someone with asthma may also have allergic rhinitis (*Bi Yuan* in CM), breathlessness (*Chuan* in CM), wheezing (*Xiao* in CM) and cough (*Ke Sou* in CM) or any combination of the above. An herbal formula would be designed around the observations the herbalist has made through the nine pulses taken on the left and right hands and tongue analysis.

For herbal treatment, I would recommend getting professional help from a qualified Qigong doctor, acupuncturist or herbalist, because treatment should be customized to the individual, which is beyond the scope of this book. Many herbalists spend their entire lives just studying herbs and their herbal actions/reactions.

Chinese Medicine also draws distinction between early onset asthma (babies and children) also called extrinsic or atopic asthma and late onset asthma. Late onset asthma, starting in adults in midlife, usually does not have such severe eczema attached to it and usually involves a completely different organ in CM. Most late onset asthma involves the Spleen (dietary problems or abuse) and the Liver (emotional problems such as repressed anger, frustration or resentment). What I am most familiar with in my case is the early onset asthma and that is what we will mostly discuss here.

Wind is usually considered the main culprit in extrinsic asthma according to CM. Wind has been a major disease pattern for thousands of years dating back to the Chinese Medicine classic the Su Wen. We aren't discussing here external wind, but the kind of rambunctious wind that gets trapped in the bronchial tubes and causes bronchial spasm. This is usually coupled with Lung and/or Kidney deficiency, which is the actual root of the disease. This, by the way, is why we discussed first that QiGong exercises strengthen these systems in order to address the root of the problem. One could like the Wind in Chinese Medicine to the western allergens, viruses or bacteria that can enter the lungs and attack the skin that we know from western medicine. In CM, the Lungs and the skin are extensions of each other, what affects one affects the other most of the time. The other factor in asthma that may seem obvious is Phlegm, but in CM it is not the cause of asthma, but a by-product that the body produces.

There are other classifications of asthma that further define the type of herbs that go into making an herbal preparation. I will only give the names of patent formulas for these conditions, as these can be bought in some of the more health conscious, progressive stores in the larger cities. The best course of action, however, is to see a qualified practitioner who can custom design an herbal preparation for you to fit your exact diagnoses in Chinese Medicine.

These are some of the herbal formulas that I have used in my practice as well as on myself. The herbalist must decide if the paramount problem stems from the eczema or the asthma in order to create the proper hierarchy of herbs in the formula. For simplicity of a complex diagnoses, I will divide the symptoms into two Chinese herbal categories for the wheezing of asthma attacks, Wind-Heat and Wind-Cold. Wind–Heat manifests itself with a spreading all over the body like a wind carrying them anywhere with red, itchy and extremely dry patches.

The Wind-Cold pattern is characterized by no sweating, breathlessness and wheezing, fever and chills simultaneously, tightness in the chest and a lack of color in the face. The patent medicine for this is called Qi Guan Yan Ke Sou Tan Chuan Wan. This formula will stop the cough and break up the phlegm and return the natural flow of Lung Qi downward alleviating the asthma symptoms.

The Wind-Heat pattern is characterized by a dislike for cold surroundings or cold drinks, food, frontal headache, a loud barking cough, a thirst that cannot be quenched, and constriction in the chest cavity. The patent formula for this is called Ding Chuan Wan, or Clear Mountain Air.

Ding Chuan Wan is a wonderful herbal that does a multitude of things. From the Chinese perspective, it strengthens the Kidney and Lungs deficient defenses, returns the descent of Lung Qi back to its normal path, tonifies the Spleen for digestion, and overall strengthens Qi.

As part of a maintenance program in between asthma attacks, an herb called Dan Shen is used in chronic asthma to move and circulated Blood/Qi in the chest. According to Giovanni Maciocia, modern research has shown this herb reduces levels of IgE immunoglobulins, which we have learned, are responsible for indirect asthma attack triggers.

Air Passages: Chinese Herbals

The strength of Chinese Medicine really comes through in its treatment of the root problems and not so much in the emergency treatment of acute attacks. I for one would still use my Albuterol inhalator at the first sign of an acute attack! And for the record, the herbals I am about to discuss can be used with Albuterol without side effects. Less frequent use of the emergency inhalator should be used as a benchmark of improvement achieved by CM therapy.

My Current Chinese Asthma Formula

One of the things I have noticed in my own treatment is that as I get older, my system seems to change and therefore my symptoms do as well. This means that I constantly have to vary my approach to keeping myself well. Yes, it is a lot of work, but one cannot put a price of time or money on one's health. This is a formula that I have developed to deal with my current symptoms. A note here: I do believe that when you have early onset asthma/eczema that you are never really "cured" but go through periods of remission or dormancy, as I like to call it. Too many things environmentally out of our control can turn the tables on us, even with the best of care, and we must be prepared to deal with them.

Here is a list of ingredients that I currently use:

- Ping Chuan Wan
- Dang Shen
- Ge Jie
- Dong Chong Xia Cao
- Xing ren
- Chen Pi
- Gan Cao
- Sang Bai Pi
- Bai Quian
- Meng Shi
- Wu Zhi Mao Tao
- Man Hu Tui Zi
- Chan Tui
- Bei Sha Shen
- Fang Feng

Understand that I do not use all of these herbs at once, and I mix and match them based on my symptoms.

Eczema and Chinese Herbals

When eczema starts at a very early age, there is a good chance that asthma will follow. According to Chinese Medicine, they have the same root cause: deficiency of Lung and Kidney defensive Qi. Again a similarity occurs in treatment of dispersing Wind from the skin as it does from the interior in asthma.

Sang Bai Pi is an herb that I have used for myself; it reduces the feelings of heat that I have from my skin when it is itchy, which translates to Damp-Heat in CM. Damp-Heat manifests as redundant patches on certain parts of the body that are inflamed, oozing and itching. Additionally, this herb moves Lung Qi downward and pulls out the heat from the Lungs. So if you are itchy and your skin is breaking out with red patches and you feel "hot," this may be one of the herbs to look for in a formula. Again, we must use herbs conjunctively for the best results.

Another herb that I have used is Bei Sha Shen. This Chinese herb is used mostly for the chronic dry skin that is pervasive with chronic eczema. It also nourishes the Lung-Yin.

From the Chinese Medicine perspective, many people who are on oral steroids or who use a lot of topical hydrocortisone creams need to realize that they are draining the Kidneys' defensive Qi system, the very thing that caused their problem in the first place. This is perhaps one of the many reasons why once someone is on western medications for a while it is very difficult to wean off of them; i.e. short term relief brings long term defeat.

The use of Chinese herbals may sound complex, and frankly it is, but it is one of the most advanced systems of natural health care available. Make sure you consult a specialist in Chinese herbals, especially if you have other outlying disease such as high blood pressure, or if you are on blood thinners, for example. Herbals are powerful in that they can do miraculous things, but if you are not absolutely sure of what you are trying to do, leave choosing them to the experts.

One other word of caution: if you are currently taking any prescription drug(s) or even over-the-counter medications for any condition, check with a doctor of Chinese medicine, or a pharmacist before self-prescribing. Since Chinese herbals are powerful enough to cause change and heal, they are also cause problems as well. Drug interaction is serious business. Don't take a chance.

FINAL THOUGHTS

In the future we may be able to control asthma through medications to a greater degree, but I know in my heart that there will always be the necessity for therapies such as mine. What is sold as a miracle drug today is recalled tomorrow or shown to have repercussions on another part of the body. Western Science has advanced so rapidly in the last 50 years. What will the next 25 years bring, and at what price? Do we accept that drug therapy is the only way, or future genetic modifications? Everyone is responsible for his or her own choices in life and can blame no other. In order to make good choices, however, we must have accurate information delivered to us. I hope this book brings you to a crossroads in your life where you can make some new decisions about your health care based on my experiences of living with asthma and allergies. At the very least I hope that it has made you *think.*

Please always question, ponder the answers you come up with and be open to trying new things. In my Kwoon (martial arts training hall) I have hanging five Chinese pictographs outlining the *Five Treatise to Becoming a Master*. This is advice for becoming a master in the martial arts, a master in your profession, mastering your own mind, or mastering your own destiny. These teachings are hundreds of years old and have been followed by many enlightened beings in the past. They are the key to becoming a master of anything, including your own fate. They also outline how to manage your health affairs.

Five Precepts to Becoming a Master

Study wide and deep.

Look for information from a variety of sources, not just one doctor or just one system of thought, but from the whole world of information, perhaps even from the most unlikely sources.

Investigate and ask.

Never cease to ask questions, even when you feel they have all been answered. Things change, advice changes, and trains of thought evolve. Flow with the Tao and never "lock" yourself into a single mode of thinking.

Fully discriminate.

Once you have collected your wide band of information, begin to throw out all that is not useful at that time. If you scatter your focus all your intent and power become diffused amongst the different paths you are following

Ponder carefully.

Use both intellect and instinct to mull over these remaining thoughts and ideas. Sit and be still with the Tao, the universe, and allow time for profound thoughts to come to you naturally; they will, but you must trust and "let go."

Study perseveringly.

Never cease to continue this process. By assuming that you have forever conquered the wisdom of your dilemma by the deeds of the past, this will lead to false illusions in the future.

In accord with this advice from these maxims, I continually change my thoughts and evolve with my asthma and allergies. I have never let them stop me from doing anything I truly wanted to do and I never will. But I must continue studying, asking, discriminating and pondering to stay ahead of this inherited gift known as asthma.

Good luck to all of you on your own quest.

BIBLIOGRAPHY

Gary F. Moring
The Complete Idiots Guide to Understanding Einstein
Alpha Books, 2000

Zhang Yu Huan & Ken Rose
A Brief History of Qi
Paradigm Publications, 2001

Swami Rama, RudolphBallentine, M.D., Alan Hymes, M.D.
Science of Breath
The Himalayan Institute Press, 1979

Leon Chaitow, Dinah Bradley, Christopher Gilbert
Multidisciplinary Approaches to Breathing Pattern Disorders
Churchill Livingstone, 2002

Joseph E. Donnelly
Living Anatomy
Human Kinetics Books, 1990

Phyllis A. Balch & James F. Balch, MD
Prescriptions for Nutritional Healing
Penguin Putnam Inc., 2000

Jerry Alan Johnson, PhD.,DTCM. DMQ (China)
Chinese Medical Qigong Therapy
The International Institute of Medical Qigong, 2000

Paul Pitchford
Healing with Whole Foods
North Atlantic Books, 1993

Frank Netter
The Netter Collection of Medical Illustrations
Havas MediMedia, 1983

Frank Netter
The CIBA Collection of Medical Ilustrations, VOl 7
CIBA-Geigy Corp, 1980

Air Passages: Bibliography

Ronald Arky, MD
Physicians Desk Reference
Medical Economics Data Production Company , 1995

Kathryn L. McCance, Sue E. Huether
Pathophysiology
Mosby, 1998

Neil Campbell
Biology
The Benjamin/Cummings Publishing Company, Inc., 1990

John J. Ratey, M.D.
A Users Guide to the Brain
Vintage Books, 2001

DharmaSingh Khalsa, M.D.
Brain Longevity
Warner Books, 1997

Pierce J. Howard, Ph.D.
The Owners Manual for the Brain
Bard Press, 1994

Candace B. Pert, PhD
Molecules of Emotion
Scribner, 1997

Lida H. Mattman
Cell Wall Defiecient Forms
CRC Press, 2001

Goldmnan, Bennett, Drazen, Gill, Griggs, Kokko, Mandell, Powell,
    Schafer
Cecil Textbook of Medicine
W.B. Sanders, 2000

The New York Public Libarary
Science Desk Reference
The StonesongPress, Inc., 1995

Eleanor Noss Whitney, Sharon Rayd Rolfes,
Understanding Nutrition
Seventh edition, West Publishing Company

Air Passages: Bibliography

Paul Pearsall, Ph.D
The Heart's Code
1998, Broadway Books

Michael D. Gershon, M.D.
The Second Brain
1998, Harper Collins Publishers

The following studies were extrapolated from Ken Sancier's Qigong database:

1. Huang, Hua. Shanghai No. 6 Peoples' Hospital, Shanghai, China [1]. Clinical applications of Chinese Qigong therapy and its mechanism. 1st International Congress of Qigong. UC Berkeley, Calif, USA. 100E; 1990.
2. Huang, Hua. China [1]. An approach to the treatment of bronchial asthmaby qigong. 1st Int Sem on Qigong. Shanghai, China. 92E; 1986.
3. Sung, yinxing [and others]. Sino-Japan Friendship Hospital, Beijing, China [1]. Role of qigong and taiji in respiratory rehabilitation.
1st World Conf for Acad Exch of Medical Qigong. Beijing, China. 101E; 1988.

RESOURCES FROM INNER STRENGTH

Videotapes

Asthma QiGong: Your Self Defense for Asthma

This video captures the power of the Pacific Ocean while demonstrating in detail the Medical Qigong exercises for asthma described in this book. This easy to follow format, paced so that you can learn comfortably, leads you through the complete 20 minute daily workout routine needed for you to take control of your asthma.

"After 3 weeks of doing this daily program, I reduced my need for my emergency inhalator by 50%"!

Scott Mettlin, asthmatic

Your Self Defense for Stress

This video filmed, with the power of nature, explains the stress cycle and how it affects your mind and body. It then clearly demonstrates the Medical Qigong exercises needed to control stress and allow your body to heal from the damaging affects of stress induced illness. The template for this video was a stress reduction program designed by Dr. Cibik for the Federal Social Security Administration. The exercises in this program was so effective and well received, that it was recommended viewing for all employees nationwide.

CD'S

Medical QiGong for the 21st Century

In this live presentation Dr. Cibik describing how breathing and pH affect everyone with autoimmune disorders. Learn how during stressful events, the pH is drastically changed, which leads to a negative domino-effect on healing.

Air Passages: Resources from Inner Strength

To order any resources from Inner Strength
please call
724-845-1041

or use the order form below;

Name:_____

Address:_____

City:_____ State:_____ Zip :_____

Please send me:

Self Defense for Stress Video $24.95
Asthma QiGong Video $24.95
Medical QiGong in the 21st Century $12.00

Shipping and handling .... add $4.95

Total: .... _____

Payment by: Check/ money order / Visa or Mastercard

Credit information:_____

Expiration:_____

Send payment to:

Inner Strength, Inc
825 Lovers Leap Road
Leechburg, PA 15656

Thank you! Please allow 4 weeks for delivery

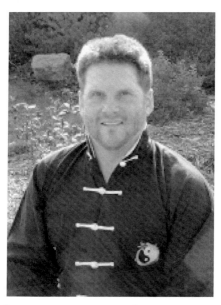

ABOUT THE AUTHOR

Ted Cibik, ND, DMQ has trained in the meditation, healing, and martial art techniques of the world since age 5. He holds multiple black belts in Kung Fu, Judo, Jiu-Jitsu and Karate. From teachers from diverse cultures, he not only learned many fighting systems, but also various healing systems and meditation systems from China, Indonesia, Japan and South America. He also studied exercise science and pre-med at the University of Pittsburgh and Pennsylvania State University and hold the title of Health and Fitness Instructor from the American College of Sports Medicine. Looking for formal education in healing, breathing and Chinese Medicine, he found Medical Qigong and graduated as one of the few Doctors of Medical Qigong (DMQ) from Beijing Western District Qigong Science & Research Institute.

In 1991, he built his 30-acre wellness facility of Feng Shui design on a mountaintop in the healing serenity of nature. Dr. Cibik believes in an integrated triune approach (physical, mental and spiritual) to health, disease management and longevity. Having treated, rehabilitated, presented to and counseled thousands of clients from around the world using a unique blend of Eastern and Western healing methods, Dr. Cibik now offers his lifetime experience and education to individuals for private and group consultation.